THE VITAMIN CURE

for Heart Disease

HILARY ROBERTS, PH.D.
STEVE HICKEY, PH.D.

Basic Health
PUBLICATIONS, INC.

The information contained in this book is based upon the research and personal and professional experiences of the authors. It is not intended as a substitute for consulting with your physician or other healthcare provider. Any attempt to diagnose and treat an illness should be done under the direction of a healthcare professional.

The publisher does not advocate the use of any particular healthcare protocol but believes the information in this book should be available to the public. The publisher and authors are not responsible for any adverse effects or consequences resulting from the use of the suggestions, preparations, or procedures discussed in this book. Should the reader have any questions concerning the appropriateness of any procedures or preparation mentioned, the authors and the publisher strongly suggest consulting a professional healthcare advisor.

Basic Health Publications, Inc.
28812 Top of the World Drive
Laguna Beach, CA 92651
949-715-7327 • www.basichealthpub.com

Library of Congress Cataloging-in-Publication Data
Roberts, Hilary.
    The vitamin cure for heart disease / Hilary Roberts, Steve Hickey.
      p. cm.
    Includes bibliographical references and index.
    ISBN 978-1-59120-264-6
  1. Heart—Diseases—Alternative treatment. 2. Heart—Diseases—Diet therapy.
3. Heart—Diseases—Prevention. 4. Vitamin therapy. I. Hickey, Steve II. Title.
    RC681.R63   2011
    616.1'2306—dc23
                                                                    2011027746

Editor: John Anderson
Copyeditor: Peggy Hahn
Typesetting/Book design: Gary A. Rosenberg
Cover design: Mike Stromberg

Printed in the United States of America

10   9   8   7   6   5   4   3   2   1

CONTENTS

ACKNOWLEDGMENTS

We would like to thank all those who have encouraged us in this work. Dr. Abram Hoffer helped create a better understanding of nutritional medicine. On this side of the Atlantic, Dr. Damien Downing, of the British Society for Ecological Medicine, has been equally helpful. Gert Schuitemaker and Elsedien de Groot have strived tirelessly to promote orthomolecular medicine in Europe. We have also welcomed the support of Dr. Atsuo Yanagisawa, a pioneer of the use of vitamin C therapy in Japan.

Bill Sardi sends frequent emails detailing developments in orthomolecular medicine, particularly vitamin C. He shows a high degree of sophistication in selecting critical papers of interest. Owen Fonorow and the Vitamin C Foundation have kept Linus Pauling's work on vitamin C and heart disease in the public eye. A stimulus for our work has been discussions with Dr. Michael Gonzales and Dr. Jorge Miranda-Massari. We would like to thank Hilary's father, Michael Roberts, a retired consultant surgeon, who discussed the conventional viewpoint with us. We are also grateful to Fiona Roberts, and to Eileen and George Fondis, for the generous loan of their computers. The macrophage cartoon is copyright by Dr Mikael Nicu of the University of Helsinki reproduced with permission.

In particular, we would like to thank Dr. Jim Jackson for his outstanding work in nutrition. His research has changed the way nutrients are viewed by the current generation of scientists.

PREFACE

A major aim of this book is not to offer medical advice but to provide a context for future research in atherosclerosis. The authors disclaim any responsibility for use of the information contained within for any purpose, including self-medication or nutrition. We do not wish to promote any therapy, or to encourage individuals to use the information in this book to go against the advice of their physician. People electing to self-treat do so at their own risk. Of course, patients may choose to bring the book to the attention of their physicians in order to help them demand appropriate treatment.

The book aims to be accessible to readers who, though intelligent, may have little knowledge of biology, chemistry, or medicine. This involves some simplification, although we have tried to avoid being inaccurate. For example, we have not differentiated between risk factors and risk markers; this slight loss of subtlety increases the readability. Readers who lack a formal scientific education can ignore the references. If the text becomes difficult because of biochemical words or jargon, please read on—these details are not pertinent to the overall story. As far as possible, we have tried to exclude jargon.

Physicians and biological scientists should find the book an easy read. We have included references for the benefit of readers who wish to follow up on the ideas presented. Often, we have cited one example, where others might have been equally valid. References

indicate additional sources of information rather than specific jus-
tification for points. In some cases, the reference provides an alternative explanation for the point being made. However, it should
be possible to validate any of the scientific statements by following the references or by an elementary Internet or library search.

CHAPTER 1

THE NUMBER ONE KILLER

*"A great doctor kills more people
than a great general."*
—GOTTFRIED WILHELM LEIBNIZ (1646–1716)

This book is about heart disease and related conditions, such as vascular disease, stroke, and diabetes. It explains the cause of the disease and how to keep your cardiovascular system healthy. Currently, people with heart disease are told there is no cure, and that their only choices are surgery and long-term treatment with drugs. This book provides another option. Atherosclerosis, the ultimate cause of most cardiovascular disease, is both preventable and reversible. We explain how simple supplements can prevent the disease and return a sufferer to good health.

Despite millions of dollars spent on research, heart disease remains one of the main causes of death in the Western world. Around the world, about three in ten people (29 percent) die of cardiovascular disease.[1] Slightly more people die from heart disease than from stroke: heart disease is the single biggest killer in the West, with stroke in third place. One in eight adults in the United States has been diagnosed with heart disease. On average, one American dies of cardiovascular disease every minute, so someone in the U.S. has probably succumbed to the disease since you started reading this chapter.

People are so used to this situation that perhaps heart disease

1

seems inevitable, but it is not. The epidemic of heart disease is a modern phenomenon. We have written this book for people who want to reduce their risk of becoming a heart disease statistic. In particular, the book focuses on alternatives to conventional approaches for prevention and treatment of these disorders, including dietary changes and food supplements. In order to understand how these might work, we first describe the development of cardiovascular disease and how this is influenced by nutritional and lifestyle choices.

Awareness of the disease mechanisms suggests methods for direct intervention and prevention. Prevailing ideas on heart disease are often misguided, so what you read may surprise you. For example, experts attribute the disease to "risk factors," which have become part of popular culture. Cardiologists assert that "we now have overwhelming evidence that high cholesterol causes coronary disease."[2] However, when asked, these doctors have failed to produce the research paper that demonstrates how cholesterol is so harmful. Other doctors claim that there is no single cause. [3] Such multi-factorial explanations are a way of disguising ignorance. We are interested in direct causative explanations, not loose statistical associations.

This book explains the underlying causes of atherosclerosis and its deadly results, including heart attack, stroke, and aneurism. Cardiovascular diseases are caused by inflammation and oxidation in the walls of arteries; this has been known for decades, but conventional medicine has apparently failed to understand the implications of this fact. The myths have entered popular culture—a television soap opera character warns against the dangers of cholesterol, while snatching a delicious bacon and egg breakfast from under the nose of a crestfallen victim. In the popular imagination, though rarely discouraged by the medical profession, this is entirely appropriate, because viewers believe that cholesterol *causes* heart disease. As we shall see, the evidence does not support this simplistic idea. To understand a problem, it is important to approach it with an open mind. This can be hard, when misinformation floods the media. Despite popular impressions, "risk factors" do not explain heart disease: the links between them and the cause of disease are tenuous. To find out what is really going on, we need to get back to basics.

One reason for medicine's failure is increasing specialization, as doctors and researchers learn more and more about less and less. Thousands of research papers are published which require the specialist expertise of a particular discipline to appreciate their full meaning. However, medical scientists rarely have the time to trawl through papers extending back over decades; it is hard enough to keep up with developments in just one field. Over-specialization can mean that underlying mechanisms remain unappreciated for long periods. To take an analogy, suppose motor mechanics were to specialize. An "autoelectrologist" would be great if you had a faulty light or a dead battery, but not if your car was leaking brake fluid or had run out of gas!

The proliferation of heart and vascular disease is a relatively recent phenomenon. Until the last century, the condition was rare, which leads us to question why so many more people are now dying from heart disease or stroke. Fortunately, the information needed to eliminate these killers is available, if we are prepared to look for it.

WHAT CAUSES HEART DISEASE?

Atherosclerosis is a disease that thickens blood vessel walls. The term *arteriosclerosis* is sometimes used interchangeably with atherosclerosis, but more often refers specifically to stiffening of the arteries. During the development of atherosclerosis, damage to the artery wall leads to localized areas of inflammation, called plaques, which can be either stable or unstable.

Stable plaques are relatively safe. They grow slowly and although they may block an artery completely, this is rare. Unstable plaques are more dangerous. These plaques are active: they can grow rapidly or they may fade and return to being relatively healthy tissue. Active plaques have a thin, fibrous cap, covering a soft core that contains fat and white blood cells. The cap helps strengthen and enclose the plaque, increasing its stability. Despite this, plaques can become acutely inflamed, causing the fibrous cover to split open. Plaques are similar to skin pimples, which can flare up and burst at any time or may quietly fade back, leaving unblemished skin.

Generally, the body is good at healing itself. If you get a cut, the blood quickly forms a clot that prevents bleeding and protects the damaged skin while it mends. Similar healing occurs if the damage is internal. When a plaque's fibrous cap is damaged, the blood vessel attempts to heal the lesion by clotting. Unfortunately, because the injury is in a restricted space, the resulting clot may block the artery and prevent blood flow. Alternatively, a fragment of clot may break off and be carried in the bloodstream, until it lodges in a vessel that is too small for it to pass. A heart attack (or coronary thrombosis) happens when an artery supplying the heart is blocked by a blood clot and the heart muscle is deprived of oxygen.

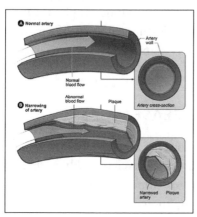

ATHEROSCLEROSIS

Sometimes a clot ends up in the brain, where the resulting lack of oxygen destroys an area of brain tissue, resulting in a stroke or cerebrovascular accident (CVA). The most common form, an occlusive stroke, occurs when a blood vessel becomes blocked (occluded), preventing blood from reaching part of the brain. Often, the clot originates from around the heart. The rarer hemorrhagic stroke is more deadly and happens when a blood vessel splits, causing bleeding into the brain. A similar process of arterial wall splitting, which is known as an aneurism, can happen in other parts of the body. The arterial wall becomes thin, blows up like a balloon, and may burst.

INFLAMMATION AND HEART DISEASE

Over the last few years, researchers have realized that inflammation is fundamental to the development of heart disease and related conditions. Inflammation is ubiquitous in damaged tissues and is triggered when the body reacts to injury or infection. Its characteristics include redness, warmth, swelling, and pain; examples include the itchy lump caused by a mosquito bite or the sensitive area around an infected tooth. If you injure part of your body, it is likely to become inflamed. Whatever the cause—heat, chemical irritation, friction, infection, or something else—the tissue responds in a similar way. It is hardly surprising that damage to an artery wall results in inflammation.

Atherosclerotic plaques are now recognized as areas of chronic inflammation, rather than inert regions of stored fat or cholesterol. As often happens, this explanation is hardly a new idea, but rather one that was known, neglected, and then rediscovered. In 1852, Rudolf Virchow, an outspoken young German scientist, drew attention to deposits of lipids (another word for fats) in blood vessel walls. Dr. Virchow, who later became the most prominent German physician of the nineteenth century, described atherosclerosis as vessel wall inflammation.

The knowledge that atherosclerosis is an inflammatory disease suggests improved methods of prevention and treatment. Indeed, many drugs currently used in the treatment of heart disease, such as aspirin and the family of drugs known as statins, have anti-inflammatory, antioxidant, or antimicrobial properties, even though they may have been prescribed for other reasons.[4] Most of the conventional risk factors for heart disease and stroke are related to inflammation and free-radical damage. Viewing heart disease and stroke in this way offers a rational approach to prevention and treatment.

ARE WE ALL AT RISK OF HEART DISEASE AS WE AGE?

The short answer to this question is no. With age, our modern populations tend to have higher blood pressure and increased risk of heart attack or stroke when compared with people in the old days or in less developed cultures. Heart attacks are largely a modern epidemic and, although atherosclerosis has existed to some extent throughout history, it only became a major killer in the twentieth century. This could reflect genetics but it is more likely a result of poor diet and lifestyle. Some older people do not develop significant atherosclerosis, have excellent blood clotting, and remain at low risk of coronary heart disease or stroke.

While most animals do not get atherosclerosis or suffer coronary thrombosis, many pet owners live in fear of a heart attack. Heart attack is a human disease, especially prevalent in those who are getting older. However, we know people who do not have this fear—they have modified their diet and now live without giving heart disease a second thought. This book offers you the chance to become one of these fortunate individuals.

RISK FACTORS

Risk factors are things that are in some way linked with heart disease. It is important to understand that so-called risk factors do not necessarily *cause* an illness, just because they are correlated with it. The term *correlated* means that variables go up and down together. For example, the number of firefighters at a fire increases with the size of the blaze; thus, we can say the number of firefighters is correlated with the fire size. Clearly, this does not mean that firefighters cause fires. Rather, the opposite is likely—the bigger the fire, the more firefighters are needed to battle the inferno.

Cholesterol is one of the most widely known risk factors for heart disease. But this does not mean that cholesterol causes heart disease and we should therefore stop eating it. It does not even mean that there is necessarily a risk associated with cholesterol in the diet. An alternative explanation is that both high cholesterol and heart disease could be caused by an unknown third variable. Confusing the association with the cause may lead to treatments that may be ineffective, if not blatantly harmful—this would be equivalent to banning firefighters, in a misguided attempt to prevent fires!

Consider another analogy. Suppose the number of reported drownings is found to increase when ice cream consumption goes up. We could jump to the conclusion that ice cream causes people to drown, and so, to save lives, we decide to ban ice cream from the seaside. (This is comparable to telling people not to eat food containing cholesterol.) However, a more likely explanation for the link is that when the weather is hot, people both eat more ice cream and swim more. Perhaps the heat drives weaker swimmers into the water to cool off, making them more likely to drown. If this were the case, banning ice cream will have no effect on the incidence of drowning. It might even make things worse, as people will be hotter without ice cream! Scientists would say "correlation does not imply causation"; it is a logical fallacy to assume that just because two factors are linked together, one must cause the other. Eating food high in cholesterol does not cause heart disease, just as intake of ice cream does not cause drowning.

A vital part of preventing heart disease is to understand the underlying biology. Blaming risk factors for the disease is bad science. Recently, many such risk factors have been proposed, often based on feeble statistical evidence. The media then discuss the importance of particular risk factors, such as eating cholesterol or watching TV. This book is concerned with cause and effect, rather than cholesterol, fats in the diet, stress, or the myriad of other conventionally suggested risk factors. However, we are unable to avoid the issue of cholesterol, so we use it throughout the book as a straw man, to illustrate the problems with corporate medicine and media hype. Despite more than half a century of research, the collected mass of details on risk factors gives little insight into the causes, prevention, and treatment of cardiovascular disease.

MECHANICAL STRESS

Plaques tend to occur in specific locations, which are mechanically stressed—often near the heart, where blood vessels pulsate, stretch, and bend. Conventional risk factors and explanations, such as high blood pressure or cholesterol, do not explain this localization of plaques within the arterial system. While most of the blood vessels are clear, those supplying the heart may be almost closed from damage and calcification.

High blood pressure and a pulsating blood flow tend to bend and twist the vessels, causing mechanical stress. The blood vessels are expanding, contracting, curving, and rotating with every heartbeat. In addition, blood flow around obstructions can cause further stress to the cells lining the artery. The blood produces a shear stress (drag) along the inner lining of the artery, where it can cause damage—rather like a river eroding its banks in a storm.

Over a single month, your heart beats about 3 million times, keeping you alive but also causing stress and damage to your arteries. Of course, minor injuries happen all the time, but the body is constantly repaired, just as the mark on your skin from a small shaving cut soon heals and fades. By contrast, inanimate objects (such as the leg of a chair) do not mend themselves, and damage builds up over time. In the case of atherosclerosis, the body's repair mechanisms eventually fail. As a result, the arteries gradually accumulate damage and scar tissue.

Mechanical stress leads to inflammation. It is easy to demonstrate this for yourself—if you rub your inner forearm hard for a while, you will see the beginnings of inflammation in the red marks that appear. If you go hiking in a pair of new boots, you may develop patches of inflammation called blisters. Similarly, inside arteries, mechanical and other stresses also lead to inflammation, stimulating plaque formation. Over time, arterial damage is inevitable, though not necessarily harmful. The plaque indicates that the body's attempt to protect and repair itself is failing and, in severe cases, a blood vessel can even rupture because of the accumulating injury. Nevertheless, a person with good repair mechanisms can live to old age without developing atherosclerosis.

OXIDATION

Mechanical stress and inflammation trigger oxidation, a biochemical process that is analogous to rusting or slow burning. The brown surfaces on toast or on slices of apple left exposed to the air are caused by oxidation. In the body, oxidation damages the cells and tissues. People take antioxidant supplements to prevent internal oxidation, which ages the body and damages its tissues. Sunlight causes free radicals and oxidation damage in the skin, leading to premature aging and wrinkles. Antioxidant face creams and sunblock are the cosmetics industry's response to aging skin.

Inside blood vessels, the oxidation associated with mechanical or chemical stress can cause white blood cells to stick to the arterial wall, in an early stage of plaque formation.[5] Importantly, this adhesion does not happen if sufficient antioxidants are present. The antioxidants in the body vary with what people eat and, to a lesser extent, their lifestyle. Tobacco smokers on a junk food diet have fewer available antioxidants than vegetarians who take antioxidant supplements. Atherosclerosis starts because of a lack of antioxidants—it is typically caused by nutritional deficiency. It is not the result of eating too much saturated fat, but of too few nutrients.

A simple "cure" for heart disease and stroke exists: with an optimal intake of vitamin C, together with other antioxidants and nutrients, people need no longer fear this disease. This idea is based on the accumulated results of decades of scientific research. The evidence suggests that freedom from these killers requires only modest dietary change. Eradication may simply require appropriate supplementation and a reduced intake of sugar.

This book explains how dietary deficiency causes atherosclerosis, which leads to coronary heart disease and stroke. The damaging free radicals are associated with tissue oxidation, which can be prevented by antioxidant supplementation. In many cases, use of high levels of specific antioxidants may reverse the disease.

IMPORTANT POINTS

- Heart attacks have a *cause.*

- Risk factors do not *cause* heart attacks (or anything else).

- Coronary disease is predominantly a human condition.

- Heart attacks and occlusive strokes can be avoided with suitable nutrition.

- Cardiovascular disease is not a normal part of aging.

CHAPTER 2

THE HEART AND CARDIOVASCULAR SYSTEM

"The best doctors in the world are Doctor Diet, Doctor Quiet, and Doctor Merryman."
—JONATHAN SWIFT (1667–1745)

The cardiovascular system is the primary transport mechanism in the body. With the heart as its pump and the blood vessels as its pipes, this intricate system supplies blood to the body tissues, delivering nutrients, hormones, and protective white blood cells. However, comparisons with central heating or automobile cooling systems stretch analogy to the limit—the cardiovascular system is far more complex. Even apparently simple biological systems are more complicated than anything constructed by human engineers, with layers of exquisitely sensitive and versatile controls.

The most critical role of the cardiovascular system is to deliver oxygen to the body tissues. Cells use oxygen to generate energy by metabolizing (burning or oxidizing) food. Without oxygen, these reactions would stop and cells would soon run out of energy—for example, brain cells die within minutes when deprived of oxygen. Paradoxically, oxygen itself is poisonous! However, our bodies depend on oxidation and reduction reactions, without which we would die.

The process known as oxidation removes electrons from molecules; its opposite is reduction, which donates electrons. Antioxidants such as vitamin C donate electrons and are known as reducing agents or free radical scavengers. Despite the body's need for oxygen and its associated reactions, it expends a great deal of energy generating antioxidants and preventing unwanted oxidation. As a rule, antioxidants are beneficial, while oxidants cause free radical damage. A free radical is simply a molecule or atom with an unpaired electron; such highly energetic free radicals can tear apart the delicate molecular structures within our cells. To prevent this free-radical attack and associated oxidation damage, cells use the energy they generate to produce antioxidants, which can neutralize the free radicals.

The importance of these oxidation-reduction reactions is illustrated by the speed with which death occurs when the cardiovascular system ceases to supply our tissues. Brain cells die within minutes. Everyone should have a basic understanding of oxidation and reduction. A simple mnemonic is OILRIG, standing for "Oxidation is Loss, Reduction is Gain" (of electrons). Too much oxidation is a feature of both aging and disease.

OXIDATION AND REDUCTION		
Antioxidant	A loses electron to B	A is oxidized
Oxidant	B gains electron from A	B is reduced

Mnemonic: OILRIG (Oxidation is Loss, Reduction is Gain)

The main cause of heart attacks, and of most strokes, is prevention of blood flow to the crucial tissues, which happens when a blood vessel is blocked by a clot. To avoid such clots, the cardiovascular system is largely self-regulating and able to repair itself. Injuries to the large arterial walls must be repaired continuously; otherwise, the damage accumulates.

If a clot prevents blood—and, therefore, oxygen—from reaching the cells, tissue damage and death will result. Cells without oxygen rapidly lose the ability to generate energy and antioxidants.

While this lack of oxygen can cause cell death, surprisingly, when the blood supply returns to the tissue, further free-radical damage occurs. The resupply of oxygen itself drives oxidation, in a process called reperfusion injury. Much of the damage in a stroke or heart attack is caused by reperfusion; additional tissue is killed when the blood supply returns to the injured tissue.

BLOOD CIRCULATION

The circulatory system consists of the heart, the blood, and the blood vessels. Humans have a closed circulation—the blood remains within its system of vessels. Introducing air into the system, which can happen accidentally while injecting drugs or through an intravenous infusion, can be deadly. The resulting bubbles can block the small blood vessels supplying the heart muscle, producing a heart attack. Alternatively, blockage of a vessel supplying the brain can cause an occlusive stroke. Other essential organs may be affected; for example, a pulmonary embolism occurs if the blood supply to the lungs is interrupted.

The pipe-work of the circulatory system separates into arteries, veins, and capillaries. A tree-like structure of arteries, ending in minute capillaries, supplies oxygenated blood to the tissues. Similarly, the capillaries drain into a sequence of veins of increasing diameter, which carry blood back to the heart. The deoxygenated blood that returns to the heart is at a lower pressure than arterial blood. Veins have thinner walls than arteries, as they do not need to withstand the high pressures needed to push the blood through the fine capillaries within the tissues of the body.

THE HEART

The heart is a four-chambered muscular pump situated in the chest slightly to the left of the midline, beneath the sternum (breastbone). In typical adults, the heart weighs about 250–300 grams. Heart muscle is highly adapted for pumping blood around the

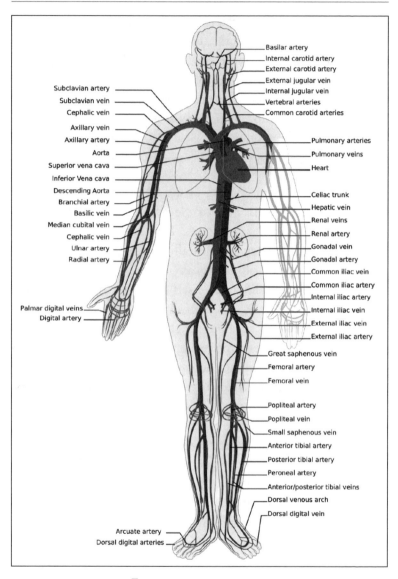

Basilar artery
Internal carotid artery
External carotid artery
External jugular vein
Internal jugular vein
Vertebral arteries
Common carotid arteries

Subclavian artery
Subclavian vein
Cephalic vein
Axillary vein
Axillary artery
Aorta
Superior vena cava
Inferior Vena cava
Descending Aorta
Branchial artery
Basilic vein
Median cubital vein
Cephalic vein
Ulnar artery
Radial artery

Pulmonary arteries
Pulmonary veins
Heart

Celiac trunk
Hepatic vein
Renal veins
Renal artery
Gonadal vein
Gonadal artery
Common iliac vein
Common iliac artery
Internal iliac artery
Internal iliac vein
External iliac vein
External iliac artery

Palmar digital veins
Digital artery

Great saphenous vein
Femoral artery
Femoral vein

Popliteal artery
Popliteal vein
Small saphenous vein
Anterior tibial artery
Posterior tibial artery
Peroneal artery
Anterior/posterior tibial veins
Dorsal venous arch
Dorsal digital vein

Arcuate artery
Dorsal digital arteries

THE HEART AND CIRCULATION

body. Unlike normal skeletal muscles, heart muscle never rests, as it must continue beating throughout life, from before birth to old age. To keep pumping blood consistently over a lifetime, heart muscle relaxes between each heartbeat.

Although we often refer to the heart as a single pump, it is actually two pumps—a right heart pump, and a left heart pump. A muscular wall called the septum divides the two. Each of the two sides is further divided into chambers: the right atrium and ventricle, and the left atrium and ventricle. The right side of the heart receives de-oxygenated ("used") blood from the body in through the right atrium, and pumps it through the right ventricle to the lungs. In the lungs, the high carbon dioxide (CO_2) content of the used blood is exchanged for oxygen, in millions of tiny, balloon-like sacs called alveoli. The alveoli are surrounded by a network of capillaries, generating a large surface area for the exchange of oxygen and carbon dioxide between the blood and air.[1] Estimates of the lungs' surface area vary, but it is often described as covering about half a tennis court!

Oxygen in the lungs diffuses through the capillary walls and into the blood, to be returned to the heart. The left atrium of the heart receives the oxygenated blood from the lungs. When the left atrium contracts, it pumps blood into the left ventricle, which then contracts and sends the oxygenated blood to the tissues of the body, completing the circuit.

The left ventricle is muscular, with walls over a centimeter thick to pump blood around the whole body. As the right ventricle pumps blood only through the lungs, less pressure and less muscle is needed. The walls of the right ventricle are usually less than half a centimeter in thickness. Occasionally, the wall or septum that separates the right and left chambers of the heart does not develop properly, leaving a hole that allows higher pressure blood to leak from the left side into the right. Unless the hole heals, or is surgically repaired in childhood, the body may reinforce and strengthen the lungs, to cope with the higher than normal blood pressure. To some extent, body tissues respond to applied stress by remodeling their structures—think of how exercise strengthens muscles and bones. When this occurs in the lungs, blood may begin flowing back through the hole from the right side of the heart to the left. Thus, the "used" blood finds its way into the left ventricle and reduces delivery of oxygen to the body. Many people live normal lives with a small hole in the heart and one explanation for migraine headaches is that they are caused by such a small hole. However, left untreated, a large hole can develop into a life-threatening condition, known as Eisenmenger's syndrome.

THE HEART'S OWN BLOOD SUPPLY

Like the other muscles and organs in the body, the heart requires oxygen and nutrients for energy. The coronary arteries supply the heart muscle with blood: the left coronary artery delivers blood to the left ventricle, and the right coronary artery brings blood to the smaller right ventricle and part of the left ventricle. Blood flow through these vessels is largely under local control. When the heart rate increases and the heart muscle needs more oxygen, local hormones—such as nitric oxide—are released to dilate the coronary arteries and increase blood flow.

In a heart attack, blockage of a coronary artery by a blood clot interrupts the blood supply to the heart, resulting in damage or death of heart muscle tissue. If the coronary blood flow is reduced gradually by atherosclerosis, collateral blood vessels may accommodate the change and provide an alternative supply. Small arteries in the heart are often interconnected, or anastomosed, and can compensate when minor blood vessels are blocked. However, the larger blood vessels are critical; there are no alternative pathways for blood flow, so blockages in the major coronary arteries are more dangerous.

Losing Control

Basic body functions such as breathing and heart rate are controlled by the autonomic nervous system without us having to think about them. The word autonomic comes from the Greek autos meaning "self" and nomic meaning "law." When the body is relaxed and using less oxygen, the heart beats slowly. The heart begins to beat faster with excitement or activity, responding to direct nerve impulses or to the release of adrenaline in the "fright, fight, flight, or frolic" response. (Prudish writers often omit the frolic part of this description, while other physiologists, wishing to shock, substitute the word fornicate, or something similar.) This automatic control allows the heart to adjust to the changing oxygen demands of the tissues.

In the absence of control signals, the heart regulates its own beating. A person may be brain dead but can still have a beating heart and a functioning cardiovascular system. This independence means that the heart will continue to pump even when not subject to external controls. When removed from the body, heart muscle cells can contract spontaneously in a steady cycle; so, for example, isolated yet still beating animal hearts can be used in experiments to test the effectiveness of drugs.

The heart's natural pacemaker is the sinoatrial (SA) node, located in the right atrium. This group of cells generates electrical impulses at intervals that synchronize the heart's rhythmic contractions. Although the sinoatrial node is the primary pacemaker, the atrioventricular node—located between the right atrium and the right ventricle—delays the signal passing to the ventricles. In this way, the atria contract first, forcing blood into the ventricles, which contract shortly after, sending the blood to the lungs from the right ventricle or to the body from the left ventricle.

Both the atria and the ventricles can be overloaded. If the heart beats too quickly, the heart muscle is unable to rest between beats and gets tired. Rates of about 200–300 beats per minute are described as a flutter. Higher rates, with irregular muscle fiber contractions, are called fibrillation. People who die of a heart attack often enter a period of ventricular fibrillation shortly before death.

Rapid beating is less dangerous in the atria than in the ventricles, as the atria are smaller, containing only about 30 percent of the heart's blood volume. The heart can supply blood satisfactorily through the pumping action of the ventricles alone. When a person is resting, their heart's pumping capacity is three or four times greater than required. Thus, someone with inadequate atrial pumping caused by an atrial flutter might not notice this until they start to exercise.

If a clot in the coronary arteries blocks the blood supply to the heart muscle, the resulting damage can lead to ventricular fibrillation. The damaged muscle deflects the impulse that regulates the heart's contraction. The signal reaches muscle fibers at the wrong time, and the heart muscle goes in to an irregular spasm. Muscle fibers contract at different rates and the heart literally writhes, like a proverbial can of worms. This seizure effectively stops the heart's pumping action. Since the blood supply for cardiac muscle itself comes from the heart, the muscle can rapidly run out of energy. Then the ventricles dilate, as their muscles relax through exhaustion. The heart has stopped and, unless the heart's beating control returns, the person is dead.

Once the heart enters ventricular fibrillation, it rarely recovers a normal rhythm. However, early electrical stimulation can "defibrillate" the heart muscle, restoring a regular heartbeat. Fans of medical programs on television will have seen this procedure, referred to as "shocking" the patient out of v-fib (ventricular fibrillation). External cardiac massage, using regular pressure applied to the chest, can occasionally provide a limited resupply of blood to the heart muscle and help revive the heart (the rhythm of the children's song *Nellie the Elephant* provides the correct compression rate, but sufficient pressure is required).[2] It may also pump enough blood to the essential tissues to allow a little extra time for full resuscitation.

BLOOD PRESSURE

Blood pressure is normally taken to mean the pressure in the large arteries. Clinically, this is often measured in the brachial artery of the arm. The units used for blood pressure are millimeters of mercury (mm Hg) and are relative to atmospheric pressure. Blood pressure is controlled by several mechanisms, including nerves and hormones, but the detailed mechanisms are not completely understood.

Systolic pressure is the peak pressure in the arteries generated by the contraction of the heart ventricles. Diastolic pressure is the lowest pressure and corresponds to the relaxation of the heart muscle. Normal ranges of blood pressure in the adult are typically assumed to be:

Systolic 90–135 mm Hg

Diastolic 50–90 mm Hg

Typical values for a healthy young adult at rest are usually given as 120 mm Hg systolic and 80 mm Hg diastolic, described as "120 over 80," though there are large individual variations. Some people have higher values, some lower, and others vary in the size of the difference between the two blood pressure readings. Furthermore, the measured values fluctuate, varying through the day. In the long term, blood pressure may also change in response to chronic emotional stress, nutrition, and disease. Children tend to have lower blood pressure, while readings in the elderly are often higher. The increase in the elderly can result from reduced flexibility of the arteries, but this is not necessarily a consequence of normal aging.

High blood pressure is often described as a risk factor for heart disease. However, hypertension is more than a statistical anomaly—it is a direct cause. The main concern with high blood pressure is the stress it places on the cardiovascular system. Blood pressure levels change with each pulse, putting mechanical stress on the arteries. In response to the increased pressure, an artery expands and then shrinks back elastically, damping the pressure wave. In many blood vessels, the movement in response to a heartbeat includes twisting and bending. Uncontrolled high blood pressure can result in an aneurism, which is when an artery balloons out, like a weak spot on a tire inner tube.

Atherosclerosis tends to occur in areas of high blood pressure

HIGH BLOOD PRESSURE AND AGING

In modern industrial populations, blood pressure often increases as we age. In that sense, the increase is normal and expected. However, it is not inevitable. Some people maintain low blood pressure throughout their lives; aging does not necessarily cause a large increase. Rather, increased blood pressure is a sign of poor long-term health and, particularly, an inadequate diet.

The pathological form of increased blood pressure occurs when it becomes more difficult for the heart to pump blood around the body. One reason for this is that the blood vessels have stiffened. As the heart beats, it sends a pressure wave out through the tree-like structure of the arteries. Large vessels lead into smaller vessels, which branch into even smaller ones. If the small vessels stiffen or contract, it takes more pressure to force the blood through them. To overcome this, the heart increases its pumping force and the peak blood pressure rises, from, say, 110 to 140 mm Hg. Additionally, stiff blood vessels do not relax as much between beats, so the resting pressure also rises, such as from 70 to 90 mm Hg. The cumulative result is an overall increase, in this case from 110/70 to 140/90 mm Hg.

Before you panic, however, you need to determine if you really do have high blood pressure. Blood pressure changes rapidly, depending on your level of activity and emotional stress. Standing up after sitting in a chair for while will temporarily increase your blood pressure. Furthermore, going to the doctor may cause your blood pressure to rise, simply because of the emotional stress of being in a clinical setting. This "white coat" effect may make it appear that you have abnormally high blood pressure when you are within the range of what is considered normal.

Fortunately, it is possible to prevent an age-related increase in blood pressure, and lower your chance of suffering a heart attack or stroke, by making changes to your diet and taking moderate exercise. Before going straight to drugs for high blood pressure, be sure to exploit dietary change.

and mechanical stress in the blood vessels.[3] Repeated stress from high blood pressure causes chronic local inflammation, generating an arterial plaque of scar-like tissue, as the body attempts to repair the damage. In healthy individuals, the day-to-day arterial damage can normally be mended. Young people and children have good repair potential. With age and poor nutrition, however, the repair mechanisms decline and damage accumulates.

BLOOD

Blood contains red and white cells and platelets, suspended in a clear yellow liquid called plasma. The white blood cells are primarily responsible for immunity, protecting the body against bacteria, viruses, and other foreign invaders that can cause illness. Red blood cells are much more numerous than white blood cells; these disc-shaped cells look like tiny squashed doughnuts and are responsible for carrying oxygen, bound to a protein called hemoglobin. Hemoglobin appears bright red when it is bound to oxygen, which is why blood at the site of an injury is red. Red blood cells are small, do not have nuclei, and are little more than sacks of hemoglobin. In most cells, the nucleus contains the majority of the DNA and is essential for reproduction and other basic functions. However, red blood cells are generated as "throw away" items, and they do not need to reproduce. Without a nucleus, these small stripped-down cells can squeeze through tiny capillaries. Red cells are by far the most abundant blood cells, consistent with their vital purpose in supplying the body with oxygen.

In addition to transporting oxygen, blood performs many other roles for the body. It supplies nutrients (such as glucose), removes waste products and distributes hormones (including insulin) that act as chemical messengers for communication between tissues. Another essential function of blood is coagulation or blood clotting, which requires platelets. Platelets are small, disc-like particles made in the bone marrow. Like red blood cells, platelets do not have a nucleus and, in fact, they are much smaller than red blood cells. The ability of platelets to aggregate and form a clot at the site of an injury can be lifesaving.

Blood Clotting

Although essential to life, clots occurring at the wrong time or place can block a blood vessel, leading to a heart attack or stroke. Abnormal blood clotting occurs when normal blood flow is disrupted. Stationary blood clots more easily than when it is flowing normally through the vessels. A thrombus is a blood clot that remains attached where it forms. In a large blood vessel, a small clot may decrease blood flow. In a smaller vessel, a similar thrombus may completely prevent blood flow, resulting in the death of the tissue it supplies. If a clot dislodges and moves with the blood flow, it is called an embolus. A large clot breaking off and floating free in the bloodstream is a serious event—this is the cause of many heart attacks and strokes.

Rudolf Virchow, a nineteenth-century German physician, first described the conditions leading to formation of a thrombus, which are now known as Virchow's triad:

- Injury to the blood vessel wall or arterial plaque

- Slowing in local blood flow, such as in an aneurysm

- Blood clotting disorders (hypercoagulability) or leukemia (cancer involving white blood cells)

Clots can form during atrial fibrillation, when the smaller upper chambers of the heart beat rapidly and ineffectively, as the blood flow slows. A recent heart attack suggests abnormal blood clotting. Additionally, long periods of inactivity—such as prolonged bed rest following an operation—can cause deep vein thrombosis (DVT). Hospital induced thrombosis is a major risk for patients. While cramped conditions in long haul aircraft can be a minor risk for DVT, the larger problem in hospitals is less widely reported.

Elastic stockings are sometimes used by passengers to prevent blood from pooling in the lower legs on long haul flights.

Scientists often look at extreme cases, called boundary conditions, to help understand the nature of a process. If a person's body were unable to make blood clots, that person would die from even a minor abrasion. The most well-known example of a deficient clotting mechanism is hemophilia, an inherited disease common among the royal families of Europe. If untreated, a hemophiliac who sustained a cut could bleed to death, because he or she lacks the ability to form a clot. The emerging hemorrhagic viruses, such as Ebola, are also characterized by extreme bleeding, which may help explain their virulence.

At the other end of the spectrum, disseminated intravascular coagulation (DIC) is a condition associated with excessive clotting, causing clots to form throughout the cardiovascular system. These clots block small blood vessels and can be so extensive that they deplete the platelets and clotting factors needed to control bleeding. As a result, tissues deprived of a blood supply can die while, paradoxically, spontaneous bleeding occurs elsewhere through lack of clotting factors. Snakebites and severe trauma can also lead to inappropriate clotting throughout the cardiovascular system. These examples show the complex and delicate nature of the mechanisms to control blood clotting.

As a result of decades of research, scientists have a good understanding of the human cardiovascular system. Despite this, many people hold the misconceived notion that, in atherosclerosis, arteries become blocked by a buildup of fat, which causes heart attacks. This is incorrect; an area of mechanical or other local stress causes inflammation. Next, further local damage and inadequate repair causes a clot to form in the inflamed blood vessel wall. Eventually, the clot breaks away and may block a coronary vessel. In most cases of coronary heart attack or occlusive stroke, the cause is a blood clot, often arising from an arterial plaque some distance away.

ARTERIAL PLAQUES

Risk factors do not explain why heart attacks are a phenomenon largely restricted to people. One of the most notable features of heart attack is that it is a disease of humans. Veterinarians do not tell pet owners to avoid feeding a high-fat or high-cholesterol diet to their cats. Cats thrive on a diet of meat and fat but rarely suffer heart attacks. In contrast, humans are prone to a form of atherosclerosis that causes widespread damage to the arteries and concentrates in arterial plaques.

Atherosclerotic plaques are an accumulation of fatty tissues and cells within the arterial wall. These walls are composed of cells, which are major players in the story of plaque development. Cells are the smallest biological objects that are fully capable of independent existence and reproduction. In our multicellular bodies, they cooperate and combine to form organized tissues. With medicine's recent emphasis on genetics, and on social and clinical sciences, cell biology tends to be ignored. However, the properties and behavior of cells generate the structure of our bodies and play a central role in resistance to disease.

Cells have many interesting and largely unappreciated properties. We think of typical cells as being microscopic, but this is not always the case. The yolk of an ostrich egg is the bulk of a single cell and, by volume, is one of the largest known cells. However, some dinosaurs had larger eggs and some nerve cells in the spinal cords of mammals can be measured in meters.

Most cells are independent living organisms. Single cells have complex behaviors and are capable of surprising feats of information processing. Some single-celled organisms can build their own homes[4] and others can find the best path through a maze![5] Cells are mobile chemical factories that can be specialized for many different functions—for example, white blood cells called phagocytes search out and destroy bacteria and engulf foreign particles, while nerve cells are responsible for transmitting electrical impulses.

Even many scientists do not fully appreciate the variety of activities of which single cells are capable. An appreciation of cell behavior aids understanding of how plaques form.

The early stages of plaque formation involve the attraction of white blood cells to a damaged site and the proliferation of cells within the arterial tissue. Atherosclerosis is not a passive buildup of waste, like the furring up of a water pipe, but an active process that depends on the response of cells to a local injury within an arterial wall. Initially, the artery may respond by thickening and expanding its wall in order to keep the blood flowing relatively freely. However, thickening of a coronary artery wall makes it less flexible and can prevent it from expanding with increased blood pressure when a person exercises; the result is a tightness and pressure in the chest, called angina pectoris. In other arteries, thickening of the walls can lead to constriction and pain in the legs, known as intermittent claudication.

Eventually, the expanding plaque begins to obstruct the blood vessel and reduce blood flow; this gradual constriction is called stenosis. In some cases, the plaque can continue to expand until it totally blocks the artery, completely preventing the flow of blood. However, relatively few heart attacks result from direct blockage by a growing plaque. Rather, most heart attacks are caused when the plaque ruptures, producing a crack or fissure in the internal wall of the artery. Blood then comes into direct contact with the damaged tissue and forms a clot, just as it would at the site of any other injury. The production of such a clot can have the unfortunate result of completely preventing local blood flow. More commonly, the clot can break off and block a blood vessel elsewhere. From this we can see that the immediate cause of a typical heart attack or occlusive stroke is a mobile blood clot. It has little (if any) direct connection to that strangely notorious molecule, cholesterol.

IMPORTANT POINTS

- The circulatory system delivers oxygen to the body.

- Stress can damage the arterial wall and cause inflammation.

- Atherosclerosis is just another name for inflammation of the arteries.

- Arterial plaques are hot spots of inflammation and oxidation.

- Atherosclerosis causes heart attacks and stroke.

- The most immediate cause of a heart attack is a clot that has broken away from an arterial plaque.

CHAPTER 3

ATHEROSCLEROSIS

*"Scientists now believe that free radicals are causal
factors in nearly every known disease, from heart
disease to arthritis to cancer to cataracts."*
—PROFESSOR LESTER PACKER

The theory that cholesterol in the diet—or even in the blood—causes heart disease is gradually being rejected, as its limitations become apparent. Experimental research has failed to confirm the hypothesis that cholesterol causes heart disease. What is not disputed is that cholesterol builds up within the walls of inflamed arteries, although this process may simply be a harmless consequence of the body trying to repair tissue damage.

Cholesterol molecules are carried in the blood as particles called lipoproteins, so named because the lipids (fats) are linked with proteins. The cholesterol in our bodies is often descibed as being of two types, depending on the proteins with which it is associated. Low-density lipoprotein (LDL) cholesterol is also known as "bad" cholesterol, and high-density lipoprotein (HDL) cholesterol is often called "good" cholesterol. LDL transports cholesterol from the liver to the tissues, including the arterial wall. Conversely, HDL does the return trip from the tissues back to the liver. The "good/bad" idea is rather simplistic: it suggests that if you have more HDL and less LDL, cholesterol will be transported away from the arterial wall.

27

The real issue in the development of atherosclerosis is not merely the presence of cholesterol. Something more alarming happens to the cholesterol that builds up in damaged arteries: it becomes oxidized and cross-linked. High levels of oxidizing free radicals accompany arterial inflammation. These damage the LDL cholesterol, in a way similar to butter turning rancid. The cholesterol within an inflamed artery is in constant danger of being oxidized.

This is the start of a vicious circle: the damaged cholesterol within an arterial wall promotes further inflammation and oxidation, and starts to form a fatty streak. This streak consists largely of oxidized LDL and similar fats, together with inflammatory substances and white blood cells. Given time, the streak becomes a plaque, composed of a fatty cholesterol-rich core covered by a fibrous cap. Smooth muscle cells migrate to the surface and multiply, laying down collagen to cover the plaque with its protective cap. Collagen is the main fibrous protein used to strengthen our tissues and bones. The protective fibrous cap increases the size of the plaque, and hence the likelihood of local arterial blockage. Fortunately, at this early stage, blockage is not usually a critical danger. By strengthening the plaque, the cap minimizes the chance of rupture and clotting, and prevents heart attacks and strokes—at least in the short term.

The process of damage runs through a consistent sequence of events. In the early stages of plaque development, oxidized protein and LDL cholesterol stick to the blood vessel wall, increasing free radical damage.[1] The oxidized fats cause inflammation, producing chemicals that poison nearby cells.[2] Oxidized cholesterol can cause blood to coagulate and promote calcification in advanced plaques.[3] Calcification occurs when calcium salts are deposited in the arteries, causing them to harden. Finally, the active plaque may rupture, shedding a blood clot that can lodge in a blood vessel elsewhere in the body and kill the individual, sometimes without any warning symptoms.

WHITE CELLS TO THE RESCUE?

Normally, white blood cells enter damaged tissues to provide protection against infection and to aid repair. Macrophages are a type of white blood cell that engulf and consume bacteria and other foreign bodies, by hunting down the intruder and wrapping themselves around it, in a process known as phagocytosis. In damaged arteries, however, macrophages can cause additional inflammation because they swallow up damaged LDL particles and accumulate cholesterol. As the plaque grows, the macrophages consume so much fat that they appear foamy when observed under a microscope. For this reason, they are called foam cells.

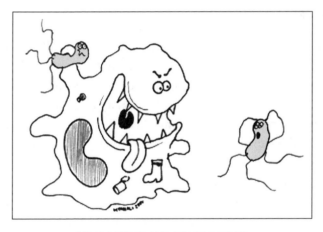

MACROPHAGE AND PHAGOCYTOSIS

The presence of foam cells indicates that the macrophages are unable to remove sufficient oxidized cholesterol and other refuse from damaged tissue. Foam cells are considered harmful and are a potential source of oxygen radicals because the absorption of oxidized cholesterol[4] can harm or even kill these white cells.[5] Unfortunately, the dying cells lead to further free radical damage and add to the deposition of sludge in advanced plaques.[6] The oxidation promoted by these cells disrupts the plaque, which can burst. The resulting clot formation may cause a heart attack or stroke.[7] Fortunately, antioxidants can help keep these white cells alive and functioning,[8] so they can continue to aid tissue repair.

Active plaques are areas of intense activity, in which the current rate of damage can overcome the body's attempts to heal itself. With time, an active plaque's inflammation weakens its fibrous cover, causing it to rupture and form a blood clot.[9] Using the example of macrophage foam cells, we can see how the body's defense system can be turned against itself. Macrophages are part of the immune system, aimed at keeping us free of infection and cleaning up detritus following injury. In arterial disease, however, something goes wrong with these normal recovery mechanisms.

SMOOTH MUSCLE

Artery walls contain smooth muscle fibers, which allow them to contract and relax, thus altering the blood pressure. Unlike skeletal muscle, which allows us to move our bodies and limbs as we wish, smooth muscle cells are not normally under conscious control. Smooth muscle tissue is controlled by the autonomic nervous system and by hormones, such as adrenaline. The autonomic nervous system controls the basic functions of tissues, such as maintaining local blood flow or the tone of muscles in the bladder. It also causes the "white coat effect" that increases your measured blood pressure in the clinic, or makes your heart pound at the thought of public speaking.

When the smooth muscle cells within artery walls contract, they reduce the diameter of the vessel to help maintain vascular tone and blood pressure, which is vital for moving blood into body tissues. If blood vessel tone is not maintained and blood is unable to reach vital organs, the body may go into shock, which can be life threatening or fatal. Even an acute emotional stress can lessen the tone and cause fainting. In this case, falling to the floor or sitting down can restore blood flow to the brain.

Arterial smooth muscle can be stimulated by mechanical stretching or by chemical or nervous signals. Stretching an artery can cause its smooth muscle to contract. These controlling influences provide the elasticity necessary to dissipate the pulsating energy of the heart's beating.[10] Smooth muscle contraction can be vital during accidental damage and trauma. If an artery is severed—for example, if a person cuts his or her wrist during a suicide attempt—the muscles in the blood vessel contract, shortening and closing the tube, to reduce blood loss and facilitate blood clotting.

In people with high blood pressure, or with atherosclerosis, smooth muscle cells may secrete local hormones and other active chemicals.[11] These chemicals attract white blood cells and act as growth promoters,[12] which can thicken the arterial wall. Muscle cells can also strengthen the developing arterial plaque.[13] As the smooth muscle cells grow, they secrete proteins that can combine with collagen and elastic fibers, forming a strengthening cover over the advancing plaque.[14] This growth of smooth muscle at the site of a plaque is initially beneficial, as it strengthens and thickens the arterial wall, preventing aneurism and bleeding.

As the plaque grows and develops, the rate of cell death in the smooth muscle tissue increases. Older cells are sensitive to additional free-radical damage and may be killed by white blood cells activated by the local inflammation. The death of muscle cells can stimulate further inflammation and oxidation, weakening the arterial wall and causing it to balloon out under pressure from the blood, forming an aneurism.[15] Unfortunately, once an atherosclerotic plaque forms, it can be self-sustaining.

PLAQUES AS INFLAMMATION

The model of heart disease as inflammation is now part of the medical mainstream. Atherosclerosis is an inflammatory disease in which plaques are active.[16] Plaques may flare up or shrink back, depending on the local inflammatory state. This explains why LDL cholesterol is a risk factor. The problems start when LDL particles collect in the internal lining, or *intima,* of the artery. This lining is formed by a thin layer of cells, together with some muscle cells, within connective tissue. Lipoprotein particles are typically able to pass into and out of this arterial lining. Sometimes, however, the LDL accumulates in the arterial wall. Surprisingly, this accumulation is not a problem in itself, as LDL is a normal part of the body and does not cause inflammation. However, when LDL enters a damaged artery, it may become oxidized or cross-linked, changing its molecular shape into a form that the immune system recognizes as abnormal. Thus, oxidized cholesterol may be a minor contributory factor to the formation of arterial plaques.

The inflammatory model of atherosclerosis, heart disease, and occlusive stroke is derived from direct experimental evidence and is consistent with the known facts. The cellular processes involved in the formation of plaques are similar to those in other chronic inflammatory diseases that involve *fibrosis,* which is the replacement of healthy tissue by scar tissue.[17] Markers of inflammation, such as C-reactive protein, are used to indicate heart attack risk in clinical practice.[18] Modern medicine is gradually accommodating this new view of heart disease.

ANTI-INFLAMMATORY DRUGS

The idea that heart disease is caused by excess inflammation suggests a possible medical intervention. Anti-inflammatory drugs are inexpensive and readily available. Could taking an ordinary anti-inflammatory such as an aspirin-like drug be the answer? Unfortunately, the answer is not so simple. First, the drug would need to enter the plaque at high concentration before it could act. It would need to be relatively free of side effects as, over time, huge quantities of the drug would be consumed. Moreover, it would have to be taken by a large fraction of the population. Even common and apparently safe drugs can cause a great number of unpleasant side effects, such as the stomach ulcers and bleeding associated with aspirin.

Aspirin is a well-known anti-inflammatory drug that is widely believed to prevent heart attacks by either "thinning the blood" or by inhibiting clot formation. In inflammatory conditions, such as arthritis, aspirin is generally taken at higher doses than those used to prevent heart attacks. It is interesting that the statin drugs, which are conventionally assumed to prevent heart attacks by lowering cholesterol levels in the blood, also have anti-inflammatory and other actions.[19] Indeed, it is unusual for a drug to have a single mechanism of action.

The cardiovascular benefits of statin drugs may arise from serendipitous side effects, rather than their intended cholesterol-lowering properties. For example, lowering blood lipids and cholesterol reduces plaque inflammation in rabbits and other animals,[20] providing an alternative explanation for the proposed benefits. These "cholesterol-lowering" drugs prevent heart attacks by decreasing inflammation, stabilizing arterial plaques, and reducing blood clotting, or by working as antioxidants. The nutritional approaches we describe later work by providing safer, long-term anti-inflammatory benefits.

OXIDATION AND FREE RADICALS

If standard anti-inflammatory drugs have limitations as treatments for heart attack, a possible alternative is to use antioxidants instead. We have seen that arterial plaques are driven by excess oxidation and free-radical damage. An understanding of inflammation leads directly to the expectation that vitamin C and other dietary antioxidants would be beneficial in heart disease.[21] Antioxidants can inhibit free-radical damage and could, in theory, prevent chronic inflammation.

The importance of these processes to health is reflected in the common use of antioxidants. To a first approximation, oxidation in a tissue produces damage, while reduction prevents it. The tissue damage caused by oxidation involves free radicals, which steal electrons from other molecules—some of which are essential substances—needed by our cells. The action of free radicals is a fundamental cause of atherosclerosis.[22] As we have explained, the free radicals released by white blood cells are a primary factor in the formation of plaques.[23] Free radicals also stimulate the increased cellular growth found in plaques. Fortunately, the free-radical reactions at the core of inflammation may be "quenched" by reducing agents. Increasing the level of antioxidants in the tissues generates a reducing environment, which helps prevent tissue damage and inflammation.

Antioxidants confer numerous benefits on heart and blood vessels. Vitamin C is required for the production of collagen, which helps to strengthen the blood vessel walls. Supplementing the diet with sufficient antioxidants can prevent lipid oxidation, and vitamin C stops LDL cholesterol from being oxidized in blood plasma.[24] Vitamin C is claimed to be an outstanding antioxidant in its ability to protect lipids in the blood from oxidation.[25] Furthermore, if a person has a heart attack or stroke, antioxidants can limit the damage caused by the reduced oxygen supply and later reperfusion injury.

One of the more recently identified risk factors for cardiovascular disease is the amino acid homocysteine. Some research has shown that high blood levels of homocysteine can damage arterial walls by producing free radicals,[26] although the evidence is not complete.[27] High levels of homocysteine may simply indicate chronic nutritional deficiency. Homocysteine is produced from the amino acid methionine, when the diet is deficient in vitamins B_2 (riboflavin), B_6 (pyridoxine), B_{12} (cobalamin), folic acid (another B vitamin), and other nutrients. People are starting to become aware that homocysteine is a "risk factor," though they are often not informed that this is the result of nutritional deficiency, particularly lack of B vitamins. Lowering the levels of homocysteine will not prevent a heart attack if something else is causing the damage. The American Heart Association (AHA) has the following statement on its website: "We don't recommend widespread use of folic acid and B-vitamin supplements to reduce the risk of heart disease and stroke. We advise a healthy, balanced diet that is rich

B VITAMINS FOR A HEALTHY HEART

The B vitamins have multiple roles in the body and they are essential for a healthy cardiovascular system. Recently, there has been an increased awareness of the role of the B vitamin folic acid in heart disease.[29] However, other B vitamins and vitamin C play an equally important role, if not more so. An inadequate intake of vitamins C, B_2, B_3, or B_{12} may mean that the arteries do not generate an adequate response to local stress.[30] The result is that stressors such as high blood pressure, rapid blood flow, and chemical attack, can injure the artery.

An abnormally high level of the amino acid homocysteine in the blood is a risk factor for cardiovascular disease. High blood levels of homocysteine are linked to damage to the internal lining of blood vessels and promote smooth muscle growth within the artery wall.[31] High levels of homocysteine are a marker of inadequate nutrition,[32] particularly deficiencies of B vitamins. Supplementing with these nutrients may be helpful in preventing cardiovascular disease and can also lower homocysteine. It is also worth mentioning that folic acid increases the synthesis of nitric oxide, an essential local hormone that may be anti-inflammatory. The effects of vitamin C are complementary to the beneficial actions of folic acid and other B vitamins, so combining the supplements may offer greater effects.

The nutritional requirement for B vitamins is increased for people who have high conventional risk factors, such as those who smoke cigarettes, have high cholesterol, or who are diabetic. Increased physiological stress, particularly oxidation, interferes with the production of nitric oxide.[33] The B group vitamins, which may alleviate this effect, are usually found together in the diet and are often taken together by supplement users. However, corporate medicine has tended to recommend either taking just folic acid or getting all your vitamins through diet alone. B-100 supplements, which contain high levels of the full range of B vitamins, are inexpensive, safe, and widely available. Rather than taking an isolated folic acid supplement, consider taking a daily B-100 to gain the full benefit.

in fruits and vegetables, whole grains, and fat-free or low-fat dairy products."[28]

Someone should tell the AHA that people often eat junk food. A person with high homocysteine is already nutritionally deficient. Few such people consume adequate diets and the reader may consider the association's advice to be unrealistic, naïve, or idealistic in its recommendations. The obvious solution is to take a low-cost multi-B-vitamin supplement, which will lower homocysteine levels. However, high-dose nutritional supplements are consistently seen as a threat to profitable drug therapies, which would be largely unnecessary with appropriate nutrition and supplements.

THE OXIDATION THEORY

The oxidation theory is an extension of the inflammatory model of atherosclerosis. It does not invalidate any of the claims for the involvement of inflammation in atherosclerosis; it simply suggests that plaques arise principally from oxidation, induced by free radicals.

An active plaque is an area of intense oxidation, which requires a large flow of antioxidants through the tissue to neutralize free radicals. While it is generally accepted that supplementing with suitable antioxidants can help to reduce plaque formation, the dietary antioxidants need to penetrate the plaque at sufficient concentration to have an effect. Many dietary antioxidants cannot do this.

A fire is an extreme example of local oxidation, so a suitable analogy for this process might be trying to quench a fire with water. In this analogy, a typical antioxidant is a cup of water. In its early stages, a cup of water may prevent a fire taking hold, but it would have no effect on an intense bonfire. Such a fire would need a fire hose or numerous buckets of water, whereas a house on fire may require thousands of gallons. Similarly, an established plaque might need massive amounts of antioxidants to quench its oxidation. The much maligned cholesterol, often blamed for atherosclerosis, merely provides material for the local oxidative fire. Furthermore, even HDL, or "good" cholesterol, can be oxidized.[34] In our bonfire analogy, cholesterol is just part of the wood pile, forming the fuel for the fire; essentially, it is harmless until lit by local oxidation.

In a healthy person, LDL cholesterol and other lipoproteins are normally protected from oxidation. People in good health have adequate levels of antioxidants. Within an atherosclerotic plaque, LDL cholesterol has limited resistance to oxidation,[35] although it does contain small amounts of antioxidants such as vitamin E and coenzyme Q_{10}. Experimentally, isolated LDL can be oxidized, but there is a lag period during which the antioxidants within the LDL protect the other constituents, such as cholesterol, from oxidation. Adding more vitamin E can increase the resistance of LDL cholesterol to oxidation. However, with prolonged exposure to free radicals, vitamin E is overpowered. It mops up the free radicals but eventually is used up, so its protective effect is limited and the LDL cholesterol becomes oxidized. Unfortunately, when a vitamin E molecule in LDL cholesterol is oxidized, it may become a free radical itself and cause further oxidative damage.[36] Even protective antioxidants have their limits and, under intense free radical attack, can become harmful.

One way of preventing vitamin E and other antioxidants from being depleted through oxidation is to take in plenty of vitamin C. Most normal dietary antioxidants do not have sufficient antioxidant power to protect against intense oxidation. However, vitamin C is a small, safe, water-soluble antioxidant that can be taken in huge doses. In high enough doses, vitamin C can help other antioxidants to remain effective.[37] The oxidized vitamin C can then be excreted in the urine and replaced by fresh supplies. Vitamin C can therefore supply the ammunition (in the form of electrons) necessary for the battle against free radicals.

In addition to aiding other antioxidants, vitamin C can prevent the oxidation of LDL cholesterol directly.[38] High levels of this vitamin can immerse the cholesterol lipoproteins in a reducing liquid

that prevents free-radical damage. However, despite ample experimental evidence for a protective effect of dietary antioxidants,
many recognized authorities still claim that they provide limited
benefit. Later, we will return to antioxidants, particularly vitamin
C and the tocotrienols, a form of vitamin E. These powerful nutrients may hold the key to preventing and reversing cardiovascular
disease.

ATHEROSCLEROSIS AND CANCER

It may sound surprising, but there could be a connection between
atherosclerosis and cancer. One idea concerning the origin of arterial plaques is that they may form in the same way as small benign
tumors. A mutation sets off abnormal cell division; the mutated
cell divides to create multiple copies (clones) of itself, forming a
lump. Such benign tumors should not be confused with malignant
cancer. A malignancy may start as a benign tumor but develops
over time into something more sinister. Cells in a malignant tumor
are a population of highly diverse cells, which differ from each
other and from the host. By contrast, benign tumors develop from
the cloning of a single mutated cell. They are common and, as the
name suggests, are usually harmless.

By 1976, it was suggested that many arterial plaques showed
clonal development of cells. In most raised plaques, a single cell
had proliferated, forming a small, localized patch.[39] The compact
nature of these patches implied they might arise from single mutated cells. Suggested mutagens included viruses and substances
derived from cigarette smoke or oxidized cholesterol. It has been
confirmed that human plaques contain cells with similar genetic
origins.[40] This suggests that arterial plaques could have a similar
origin to that of a benign tumor. The similarity between arterial
plaques and early-stage tumors was made more explicit when it
was found that the DNA in plaque from two different animals had
similar genetic changes to those expected in some tumors.[41] This
is not surprising, as both are examples of abnormal growth.

Despite this similarity, it is not clear that plaques originate as benign tumors. The arteries themselves are constructed from patches of cloned cells. During development, a single cell multiplies and generates a small local section of an arterial wall. It is therefore possible that promoting the growth of cells in a small section of arterial wall would generate clones.[42] The similarity of the cells in a plaque could simply indicate that it is derived from a particular area of arterial wall. However, noting the similarity between a plaque and a tumor highlights that they both involve cell division and growth. The development of an arterial plaque, by a mechanism in which the artery wall responds to insult or damage, may have a fundamentally similar origin to that of a cancer.[43] If early cancer and atherosclerosis do indeed develop by similar mechanisms, it implies that interventions that reduce the risk of one disease may also inhibit the other.[44]

By preventing free radical damage, antioxidants can stop mutations and abnormal cell growth. Most forms of damage to our cells involve free radicals—for example, when an x-ray causes a mutation by generating free radicals that attack a cell's DNA. It is slowly becoming clear that both cancer and atherosclerosis involve oxidative damage by free radicals, as well as inflammation and angiogenesis (the promotion of local growth of blood vessels).[45] These processes are all influenced by diet and nutrition. Good nutrition benefits the whole organism and can prevent or mitigate the effects of more than one chronic disease. There is thus a good chance that taking antioxidant supplements to protect against cardiovascular disease may also lower your risk of cancer.

A CLUE FROM TRANSPLANT FAILURE

Observations from organ transplant patients suggest that many current ideas about heart disease are wrong. Atherosclerosis is not necessarily a long-term disease arising from multiple risk factors. It may happen quickly and can be an acute problem, even in the young.

Perhaps surprisingly, the leading cause of death in the first year after a heart transplant is atherosclerosis, which may be rapid and aggressive. Similarly, cardiovascular disease is the most common cause of death following a kidney transplant, carrying an annual risk of about one in twenty patients, which is about fifty times the number in the general population.[46,47] During a transplant operation, the recipient's blood vessels are connected to those of the donor organ. However, the vessels may have different diameters, causing a discontinuity and partial obstruction to blood flow where they join. Furthermore, scar tissue at the the attachment site forms a stress hotspot, as it is stiff and less resilient. The problem appears shortly after transplantation and impairs the arteries' ability to expand and respond to fluctuations in blood pressure. In short, organ transplants involve severe local arterial damage.

Damage to the arteries following an organ transplant accelerates atherosclerosis and generates transplant vascular disease (TVD). As might be expected, the conventional explanation is that many factors are involved, implying that researchers are employing a standard scattergun approach and covering all bases.[48] Suggested factors for TVD include:

- Pre-existing atherosclerosis made worse by surgical trauma.

- Oxidation damage as a result of reperfusion injury when the blood supply is reattached to the transplanted organ.

- Lack of a nerve supply, which reduces arterial responsiveness.

- Damage to the lymphatic system that drains fluid from the organ.

- Immune disruption, activated by the transplant or by suppression with anti-rejection drugs.

- Traditional risk factors for coronary artery disease, including high blood fats, diabetes, high blood pressure, and so on.

- In kidney transplant patients, a higher oxidation status than healthy controls may contribute to inflammation.[49]

- Finally, microorganisms, such as herpes viruses, may be involved.

Several of the factors suggested above provide information about the progression of the disease, without clearly specifying the cause. Conventional risk factors do not explain the rapid onset of atherosclerosis. Atherosclerosis in transplants probably results from inflammation, due to mechanical damage that is not properly repaired, as well as from the inflammatory actions of anti-rejection drugs. The unfortunate finding that children who receive transplants also suffer atherosclerosis is a brutal fact, which highlights the inadequacy of the multifactorial approach.

IMPORTANT POINTS

- Atherosclerosis occurs when the arterial wall cannot repair itself.

- Damage builds up over time, producing chronic inflammation.

- Organ transplants and surgery to the arteries can produce rapid local atherosclerosis.

- Even children who have had transplant surgery can develop rapid onset atherosclerosis.

CHAPTER 4

A BIG FAT LIE

"Great theories are expansive;
failures mire us in dogmatism and tunnel vision."
—STEPHEN JAY GOULD, *EIGHT LITTLE PIGGIES*

The cholesterol story is so widespread that we need to begin by addressing the question raised by science writer Gary Taubes: what if it's all been a big fat lie?[1] Although the belief that dietary cholesterol causes coronary heart disease has been popular with the medical community and the media for over half a century, it is essentially a myth. Cholesterol is essential to our bodies—it is manufactured in the liver and is in every cell. Cholesterol is particularly vital for healthy brain function: too little cholesterol will cause illness, such as depression.[2] It could even increase the likelihood that a person will commit a violent crime.[3] For women over fifty, low cholesterol is associated with increased risk of death from cancer or liver disease, and with mental illness.[4] Elderly patients who go into hospital with low cholesterol are at greater risk of death than those with higher levels.[5] Severely ill patients and those in intensive care often have low cholesterol and lipid supplementation has even been suggested as a treatment.[6] Intensive care patients with low cholesterol levels are at increased risk of death, compared to those with higher levels.[7] Generally speaking, whether you are elderly or you are an adult in good health, if your cholesterol is too low, you are at greater risk of illness and death.

43

So, if cholesterol is vital to health, why has it gained such a bad reputation? One reason is that it is found in arterial plaques, which has led researchers to conclude that it plays a part in the development of heart attack and stroke. Unfortunately, the overwhelming emphasis on research into cholesterol over recent decades may have delayed progress in understanding these diseases. Cholesterol research has generated a long series of publications which throw little light on the problem of heart disease. Coincidentally, the focus on cholesterol creates the impression that the idea has obvious value or else so many doctors would not be working in this field. The recent clinical literature on cardiovascular disease has been dominated by research into the cholesterol-lowering statin drugs.

The widespread and popular misunderstanding of heart disease is that cholesterol builds up on the surface of arterial walls, ultimately blocking the artery and causing a heart attack or stroke. According to this model, the root cause of the problem is believed to be too much cholesterol from a high-fat diet, circulating in the blood and building up inside the arteries. Until quite recently, the conventional medical explanation was rather similar. However, although high blood cholesterol may indeed be a "risk factor" for heart disease, so are many other aspects of our diet and lifestyle. Critics of the idea cite compelling evidence that people with normal or even low blood cholesterol have heart attacks. Furthermore, there is little to link *dietary* cholesterol to *high blood levels* of cholesterol.[8] Those dreaded cholesterol-laden eggs are a healthy part of the normal diet. The much-maligned butter is preferable to the overhyped and allegedly healthy margarine.

The case against the cholesterol myth has been detailed by Dr. Uffe Ravnskov[9] and others, who point out that high blood cholesterol is not closely associated with atherosclerosis found during postmortems. Blood cholesterol is also not correlated with the results of coronary angiography, which is an x-ray examination of blood vessels in the heart. As we explained earlier, established plaques contain calcium deposits. The buildup of calcium deposits in older arterial plaques, called calcification, is due to chronic inflammation, and is not the result of high levels of cholesterol in the blood. In addition, atherosclerosis in peripheral blood vessels is not closely linked to high levels of blood cholesterol.

BEGINNINGS OF A MEDICAL MYTH

Felix Marchand introduced the term *atherosclerosis* in 1904, proposing that it was the cause of obstructive artery disease.[10] It was noted that atherosclerotic arteries contained abnormally large amounts of cholesterol.[11] The cholesterol story began soon after, early in the twentieth century, when it was suggested that there might be a connection between fatty foods and heart disease.[12]

In 1913, Nikolai Anichkov carried out experiments on rabbits, which led him to claim that cholesterol alone causes atherosclerotic changes.[13] He fed rabbits on purified cholesterol dissolved in sunflower oil and found they developed fatty streaks and deposits of cholesterol in their artery walls. The more cholesterol they consumed, the more deposits they developed. Control rabbits, fed only on sunflower oil, did not show the same changes. Anichkov therefore concluded that cholesterol causes atherosclerosis. William Dock, reviewing the first fifty years of research into atherosclerosis, claimed this "classic" work was one of the major developments in medical science.[14] Likewise in 2002, the lipid hypothesis of heart disease was hailed as one of cardiology's ten greatest discoveries of the twentieth century.[15]

Despite this acclaim, the results of Anichkov's experiments were not as conclusive as he and his followers had supposed. Regardless of what these experiments tell us about rabbits, humans are different and extrapolation from one to the other is risky. To begin with, the benign fatty streaks Anichkov observed in rabbits differed greatly from the dangerously unstable plaques found in human atherosclerosis. Later research has shown that considerably more effort is needed to produce human-like plaques in rabbits. In addition to a cholesterol-rich diet, the procedure involves mechanical trauma to the artery (produced by inflating a balloon within it), followed by injections of histamine (to enhance inflammation) and viper venum (to stimulate blood clotting).[16] If cholesterol really caused plaques, these interventions would not be necessary. Humans and rabbits have contrasting dietary needs: rabbits are herbivores—they live on a low-cholesterol diet of vegetation and are able to produce vitamin C in their bodies. In their natural habitat, they do not develop the form of heart disease found in humans. The so-called atherogenic (atherosclerosis-producing) action of cholesterol is inhibited by the rabbits' naturally high internal production of vitamin C. Rabbits do not get heart attacks when fed a high cholesterol diet. Humans, by contrast, are omnivores and, although they cannot produce vitamin C internally, they have adapted to a diet rich in cholesterol and other animal fats. There is little evidence either that rabbit plaques are equivalent to human ones or that these experimental findings from rabbits apply to people.

In the early to mid-twentieth century, the number of people dying from heart disease increased by a factor of about ten. Previously, some people developed atherosclerosis, but few died from heart disease.[17] Ancel Keys, a scientist from the University of Minnesota, thought he knew why.[18] In the early 1960s, Keys described three factors he believed were associated with risk of heart attack: smoking, high blood pressure, and cholesterol.[19] On a trip to a conference in Italy in 1951, Keys learned that coronary heart disease was not a major problem locally. He found that blood cholesterol levels in Italians were lower than those in the United States and assumed that this was because Italians consumed less saturated fat, such as that found in butter or milk, and more unsaturated fat, such as that in olive oil.[20] Later, Keys found that the blood cholesterol levels of Japanese migrants to the United States gradually increased, which he attributed to their change in diet.[21] Keys believed he had discovered that reducing the amount of saturated fat in the diet lowered the amount of cholesterol in the blood.[22]

Keys' ideas seemed to be confirmed by studies of death rates in Norway during World War II. Food shortages were apparently linked with a decrease in the death rate from both heart disease and other factors.[23] However, life before the war was different to how it was during the hostilities in many ways, beyond the consumption of saturated fat. Any of a large number of factors might relate to the observed decrease in heart disease. In the Korean War, by contrast, the U.S. military found that their young male casualties, average age twenty-two years, had clear signs of atherosclerosis. The facts did not support Keys' suggestions.[24] Keys' risk factors could not explain the rising incidence of the disease in these young soldiers. Army rations, as used in the Korean War, had changed little since the 1880s.

In 1957, the American Heart Association reviewed Keys' conclusions about cholesterol and found them wanting. With time, the damaging effect of his other two factors (smoking and high blood pressure) on the arteries was clarified; clear and direct mechanisms exist to explain the damage. But the connection with cholesterol remains weak. Saturated fat in the diet may contribute in some vague and minor way to a heart attack, but it clearly does not cause heart disease directly. Keys' ideas did not provide an explanation for the principle features of hearts attacks which are caused by damage to the arteries and inappropriate blood clotting, rather than by cholesterol blocking arteries.[25]

These setbacks did not stop Keys. Shortly after, he and a supporter joined the American Heart Association committee on dietary fats and heart disease, which subsequently reversed its conclusions.[26] There are apparently at least two ways to make progress in medical science: one is to generate robust, reproducible data, which provides convincing evidence. A second is to join the relevant committee and persuade them to sanction your poor-quality ideas!

The idea of restricting dietary fat intake to prevent heart disease gained popularity in the 1960s, partly because of worries about the safety of anti-clotting agents, such as warfarin. As explained by

RAT POISON FOR
ABNORMAL CLOTTING?

Warfarin is a widely prescribed anti-clotting drug. As popularly described, it "thins" the blood, inhibiting clotting by blocking the action of vitamin K. Preventing abnormal clotting can lower the risk of heart attack, deep vein thrombosis, and occlusive stroke (when a blood vessel supplying the brain becomes blocked). But vitamin K does more than aid in blood clotting: it is directly involved in calcium metabolism and in maintaining healthy bones,[27] and it helps prevent arterial calcification.[28]

People on warfarin for blood clotting may find that calcium is deposited in their arteries, worsening their cardiovascular disease. Warfarin also lowers bone density, potentially leading to fracture or osteoporosis. Equally alarming, before becoming available as a medicine, warfarin was used as a pesticide. It is still used to kill rats, mice, and other rodents, though some pests have gradually become resistant to it.

People with abnormal clotting mechanisms need medical support, monitoring, and control. This is not an area for do-it-yourself medicine. Aspirin is often used for mild clotting disorders, but warfarin is the standard drug for severe abnormal clotting. Unfortunately, the toxicity of warfarin makes its use as a drug rather difficult.[29] Patients need to have their blood clotting carefully monitored—too little warfarin will not eliminate the risk of abnormal clotting; too much of the drug can cause dangerous bleeding.

People taking warfarin for deep vein thrombosis (DVT)[30] need to balance the risks of treatment against the benefits. About one in forty-five patients (2.2 percent) will experience a major bleed, and of these, about one in eight will die. For each year a person is on warfarin, they have a one in fourteen chance of being hospitalized as a result of abnormal bleeding. Each year, strokes occur in one of every eighty-seven patients taking warfarin. The initial three months of treatment is particularly dangerous: in the early stages of treatment, warfarin can increase clotting and, in rare cases, this causes gangrene. This reinforces the need to manage blood coagulation treatment, with regular blood testing under medical supervision.

Even if the warfarin dose is closely monitored and controlled, there are other dangers, including possible drug interactions with many prescription and over-the-counter medications, such as statins and aspirin. Some herbs and supplements, such as garlic, need to be avoided. Alcohol can also cause problems. Even foods that contain vitamin K (leafy greens, such as broccoli) can affect the warfarin's activity. People on warfarin need to take extra care and many activities may need to be curtailed because of the risk of bruising or other bleeding.

In many cases, there are safe, natural alternatives to warfarin. Fish oil supplements taken at 2,000 milligrams or greater daily will increase clotting time and enhance the effects of warfarin. This is normally considered an adverse effect, but supplementing with fish oil could equally be viewed as a means of replacing warfarin treatment or at least lowering the dose.[31] By blocking the action of vitamin K, warfarin can have a stronger clinical effect than high-dose fish oil and supplements. However, the advantage of fish oils is that they have numerous positive effects on the cardiovascular system, such as preventing inflammation.[32]

Many other supplements can increase clotting time, including vitamin E, ginger, and *Ginkgo biloba*. Nattokinase, a food supplement derived from fermented soybeans, is being promoted as an alternative blood thinner to daily aspirin.[33] Nattokinase has not been fully tested clinically, but it may be effective.[34] Taken with pine bark extract, nattokinase has been found to prevent DVT on long-haul flights.[35] However, there is at least one report of a brain hemorrhage from its use along with aspirin.[36] Despite the reports, one problem with nattokinase is that it is an enzyme; as a general rule protein molecules are broken down in the gut and are thus ineffective when taken orally.

Doctors warn against natural anticoagulant supplements because of perceived risks, such as the possibility of causing excess bleeding in surgery, for example;[37] however, they do not highlight the potential benefits of such supplements. This logic is suspect. If fish oil or other supplements can lower a person's prescribed dose of warfarin, they might also decrease the incidence of dangerous side effects. In some cases, supplements may be insufficient, but many people might be able to achieve a target clotting time with supplements alone. Rather than asking people on warfarin to forgo such supplements, physicians could adjust the warfarin dose to the desired level in combination with a controlled intake of fish oil.

Sir John McMichael, FRS, Professor of Medicine at the Royal Post-graduate Medical School in London, in the *British Medical Journal*, " . . . the treatment [with warfarin] even in first-class centers is difficult to control and supervise. Serious, or even fatal, bleeding may occur in 10 percent of cases: strokes from cerebral hemorrhage are real risks. Further, those who die of the treatment are not necessarily those who would have died without it. *The regime thus involves human sacrifice for a very dubious gain.*"[38]

Although anti-clotting agents reduce the risk of heart attack and occlusive stroke, this comes at a price: they require constant monitoring of blood levels and also increase the risk of brain hemorrhage or other types of bleeding.[39] A stroke from bleeding is often more damaging than one caused by a clot. Consequently, anticoagulant treatment for heart disease was discarded for about twenty years, though recently it has come back into fashion.[40] The natural alternatives to warfarin are nutritional supplements, such as fish oils and high-dose vitamin E. The main side effects are improved health. Whenever practical, mild clotting disorders should be addressed with nutritional supplementation.

Many scientists have recognized the lack of evidence connecting cholesterol to heart disease. However, the juggernaut of such a popular myth is reinforced by its high media profile, the social climate, and continuing reports of risk factors. Doctors gain rewards rather than censure for advising patients to lower the amount of saturated fat in their diets. Furthermore, researchers have received lavish funding for decades, in an attempt to establish a role for dietary fat in heart disease and demonstrate the effects of cholesterol-lowering drugs. In such an environment, it is easy to miss or ignore books and scientific papers that present conflicting evidence.

When a sixty-year-old person's probability of a heart attack increases from 0.10 percent to 0.11 percent, this is not a major concern, considering other daily health risks. Anyone could be involved in an automobile accident, fall from a ladder, be diagnosed with cancer, or face a myriad of other possible misfortunes. However, for a large population of 300 million, this small risk might mean 30,000 extra deaths. Governments and corporate medicine are concerned with these big numbers, though they are irrelevant to individuals.

Surprisingly, what is perceived as being good for society might not be good for you personally, although what is good for the health of each individual will eventually add up to benefiting the population. Do not be fooled by the media reporting that the latest statin drug will lower your risk of heart attack by 25 percent. This apparently large percentage may be of negligible importance to you as an individual, say a decrease in your risk from 4 in 10,000 to 3 in 10,000. The promoters want to sell you the drug, not save your life.

In the 1960s, the decision to overlook inflammation and blood clotting in heart disease left the cholesterol hypothesis as the main contender. Since that time, numerous clinical trials and epidemiological studies have confirmed that smoking, high blood pressure, and cholesterol are risk factors. But a risk factor in a clinical trial does not necessarily have any practical importance for an individual.[41]

DIFFERENCE BETWEEN A RISK FACTOR AND A CAUSE

- A cause is directly responsible for the disease.
- A risk factor is in some way associated with the disease.

Example 1: As in the earlier example, suppose the number of people drowning in the sea is highly correlated with the sales of ice cream. Ice cream consumption is thus a risk factor for drowning. However, eating ice cream does not cause drowning. The observed association is because people both eat ice cream and swim more frequently when the weather is hot. The cause of drowning is water in the lungs, which stops the person being able to breath.

Example 2: Suppose people who consume a diet high in saturated fat are more likely to have a heart attack. Saturated fat consumption is thus a risk factor for heart attacks. However, saturated fat does not cause heart attacks. Modern diets that are high in saturated fat often contain large amounts of sugar and are low in nutrients, leading to chronic inflammation and blood clots. The *cause* of a heart attack is a blood clot (often arising from an atherosclerotic plaque) that blocks a coronary artery.

GOOD AND BAD CHOLESTEROL

As evidence accumulated and the limitations of the standard cholesterol hypothesis became apparent, researchers gradually modified their ideas. The main development was the distinction between "bad" low-density lipoprotein (LDL) cholesterol and "good" high-density lipoprotein (HDL) cholesterol. It is worth noting that the cholesterol molecule in these two forms is identical—it is the packaging that is different.

A popular theory about cholesterol is that excess LDL cholesterol is to blame for atherosclerosis. According to this hypothesis,

LDL accumulates in the wall of an artery where it undergoes chemical changes, particularly oxidation, resulting in atherosclerosis. However, measurements of total cholesterol levels may be deceptive. There is more than one type of LDL cholesterol and the different forms have different properties. As a result, studies linking LDL to heart disease may be confusing.

Some large LDL particles, called VLDL (very low-density lipoprotein), are considered safe, as they are too large to enter and accumulate in the arterial walls, so they remain in the bloodstream. By contrast, smaller LDL particles can squeeze between the cells and into the artery wall, where they may become oxidized. As a result, a refinement of the "bad" cholesterol idea applies the term specifically to the small LDL particles, which consequently are referred to as "bad bad" cholesterol, with VLDL labeled as "good bad" cholesterol!

Cholesterol Tests

Beware cholesterol tests. A test may tell you the total amount of cholesterol in your blood, including "good" HDL cholesterol, as well as the different types of LDL cholesterol. A person interested in his or her cholesterol levels might prefer to know the ratio of HDL to LDL cholesterol. The aim is to have higher levels of HDL and lower levels of LDL. A test of total cholesterol will not reveal this ratio, nor will it show the relative proportion of HDL to small LDL particles, which (we are told) is particularly relevant.[42] One approach is to ask your physician or the laboratory to test for triglyceride levels. High triglyceride levels are unhealthy, as they are associated with high levels of small LDL particles ("bad bad" cholesterol) and low levels of HDL ("good" cholesterol). Even doctors are becoming confused with this changing and increasingly perplexing advice.

Inappropriate medical screening is harmful. As we enter middle and old age, we are often advised to have health checkups to help avoid heart disease. People are familiar with having their automobiles routinely serviced as parts wear out. However, unlike inanimate mechanical parts, a person's tissues are self-repairing. Unless you have a strong reason to suspect you are at particular risk of heart disease or stroke, such testing may ultimately harm your health rather than protect it.[43] As a general rule, it is wise to avoid most screening tests, unless there is a good reason to suspect you have an illness. Health professionals providing the tests often do not understand the intricacies of test interpretation and will over-interpret results. A more effective approach is to maintain a healthy lifestyle, which includes eating a good diet.

FEEDBACK CONTROL AND EATING EGGS

By now, you should be aware of the lack of evidence that heart attack (coronary thrombosis) or stroke is caused by cholesterol in the diet. Moreover, dietary recommendations are tending to shift from focusing on cholesterol to other fats. The idea that including high-cholesterol foods in the diet is dangerous ignores a basic control mechanism in physiology: negative feedback. In biological systems, the term used for such feedback control is *homeostasis*. An everyday example of negative feedback is the climate control mechanism in a home. If the temperature rises above the setting, the air conditioning automatically switches on, lowering the temperature. At the desired temperature, the air conditioning switches off. In the same way, if the temperature falls below the chosen setting, the heater comes on. Similar homeostatic mechanisms exist throughout biological systems; for example, they keep your body temperature relatively constant and control factors such as the number of red blood cells in your body, the thickness of your skin, and many others.

Blood cholesterol levels are also controlled by feedback. Cholesterol enters the system in two ways—it can be consumed in our food or it can be manufactured in the liver. The liver can also break down unwanted cholesterol. Because of this, in most people, eating cholesterol in food has only a small effect on blood levels. If too much cholesterol is taken in the diet, the liver can either reduce its output or increase cholesterol breakdown. Both these mechanisms regulate the amount of cholesterol in the body. If your body's cholesterol levels are too high, it is not that you are eating too much cholesterol, but rather that the control mechanism is not working properly.

Lowering the intake of dietary cholesterol may reduce blood levels slightly, but greater production by the liver will compensate. But don't let this worry you—despite the bad press, cholesterol is really one of the good guys. It is essential to life and is made in large amounts (80 percent) by the body, with the remainder (20 percent) coming from the diet. Every cell in the body needs cholesterol for its normal structure and function. It is also used in the manufacture of steroid hormones, such as estrogen and testosterone, and in bile salts, which help us digest fats. Cholesterol deficiency is rare, but can lead to devastating complications, especially in the central nervous system, as the brain contains high levels and is particularly dependent on cholesterol.

Only an abnormally excessive intake of cholesterol over an extended period would overwhelm the body's control mechanisms. High levels of cholesterol in the blood indicate defective internal controls, rather than too much cholesterol in the diet. As long as the control mechanisms are working, there is no need to avoid eating cholesterol-rich food, such as eggs, on the vague grounds that they might contribute to heart disease.

CHOLESTEROL IN THE BLOOD

So far we have seen that there is only a tenuous link between the cholesterol in the food you eat and the levels in your blood. In addition to this, there is no direct connection between blood cholesterol levels and heart attacks. Michael Brown and Joseph Goldstein won the Nobel Prize in Medicine for their work on the body's regulation of cholesterol. They found that white blood cells called fibroblasts, which are involved in wound healing and are found in arterial plaques, have LDL receptors that enable the cells to recognize and take up "bad" cholesterol, removing it from the blood.

Brown and Goldstein were studying severe familial hypercholesterolemia, a genetic condition in which blood cholesterol levels can be five times higher than normal. They found that people with this rare disease lacked LDL receptors, so their cells did not recognize high levels of cholesterol. Thus, their bodies were not able to remove excess cholesterol from the blood effectively. In our climate control example, the problem is equivalent to the air conditioning not switching on when the temperature goes up.

People with a double dose of the defective gene have no LDL receptors—they have massively high blood cholesterol levels (five times the normal values) and can die from atherosclerosis before reaching adulthood. People who inherit only one gene for the disease have half the expected number of functioning LDL receptors, thus their blood cholesterol levels are intermediate between those who lack two genes and normal individuals. Typically, those with a single faulty gene develop atherosclerosis at around 35–55 years of age. Importantly, the plaques in patients with hypercholesterolemia are not the same as those found in common heart disease.[44] This difference should have acted as a warning to those assuming high cholesterol was the cause of the modern epidemic.

The clear link between hypercholesterolemia and cardiovascular disease seemed conclusive to many people, who thought that the elevated blood cholesterol in hypercholesterolemia *caused* atherosclerosis and death from heart attack and stroke. However, it turned out that they were jumping the gun—the deaths do not directly result from the high blood cholesterol. Indeed, the pattern of deaths from heart disease in families with hypercholesterolemia is similar to that in the general population.[45] Even massively high blood cholesterol does not necessarily cause heart disease. In the nineteenth century, the total death rate of people with hypercholesterolemia was *lower* than that of the general population. This fact refutes the idea that high blood cholesterol causes heart disease. Although high cholesterol may prevent death from other causes, the effect is not large. Despite having abnormally high levels of blood cholesterol, people with hypercholesterolemia do not inevitably suffer atherosclerosis, heart disease, or stroke.

One reason the association between hypercholesterolemia and heart disease was noticed was that if these patients had heart complaints, they were likely to be identified as having hypercholesterolemia. Cholesterol testing is standard practice for those with symptoms of cardiovascular disease. By contrast, otherwise healthy people—who were hypercholesterolemic but had experienced no cardiovascular problems—simply went unnoticed. For this reason, the connection with heart disease appeared stronger than was actually the case.

Historically, atherosclerosis seems to have been with us in some form since at least ancient Egyptian times.[46] However, actual heart attack has been relatively rare until recently. After 1915, the death rate from heart disease among both people with hypercholesterolemia and the wider population increased. It reached a maximum during the 1950s, after which it began to decrease. Clearly, something other than cholesterol was at work, causing this rise and fall in the death rate from heart disease. This is a strong indication that some environmental factor plays a causative role.

We can see why the idea that "bad" cholesterol in the blood causes atherosclerosis was so persuasive. People with hypercholesterolemia have enormously high levels of blood cholesterol and appeared to die early from complications of atherosclerosis. It was easy to assume that the excess LDL cholesterol in the blood might accumulate in the artery walls. By analogy, researchers assumed that heart disease in normal people might result from high blood levels of LDL cholesterol. However, wishful thinking is not an explanation.

If the cholesterol hypothesis were true, then controlling blood cholesterol would prevent heart disease. In science, however, the aim is to show that an idea is wrong, rather than trying to find evidence to support it. If the cholesterol theory were correct, people with low cholesterol would never get the disease. Unfortunately, they often do, and this finding contradicts the hypothesis.

STILL WANT TO LOWER YOUR CHOLESTEROL?

After reviewing the evidence, suppose you still want to lower your blood cholesterol. Perhaps your doctor has recommended that you take statins. In that case, you might consider making dietary changes and taking nutritional supplements, rather than beginning a lifetime of daily drugs, risking side effects and incurring financial costs. While cholesterol is not the cause of atherosclerosis, it is probably a minor contributory factor in the progression of the disease. There are several ways a person can manage his or her blood lipids without drugs.

Drugs

Corporate medicine suggests the use of statin drugs, which inhibit cholesterol synthesis, to lower blood lipid levels. However, once you are prescribed statins, you may need to take them for the rest of your life and even then they may not lower your risk of death from heart disease. Additionally, statins have a range of other potential side effects, including kidney, muscle, and nerve damage.[47] The drugs may cause a deficiency of coenzyme Q_{10}, which is an essential cellular antioxidant and a popular supplement.[48] As a precaution, people who decide to take statin drugs to control blood lipids are advised to take at least 200 milligrams of coenzyme Q_{10} a day. Vitamin D supplementation is also advisable, since it may help prevent statin side effects, such as muscle weakness and pain.[49]

When a doctor or researcher thinks that lowering cholesterol will prevent heart disease, they will look for a drug to do this. If such a drug does prevent heart disease, it will be taken as confirmation that cholesterol causes heart disease, even if the result was pure luck or unrelated to the drug's cholesterol-lowering action.

Cholesterol-lowering drugs often have many other effects.[50] For example, they may inhibit inflammation[51] or act as antioxidants,[52] both actions that can protect against atherosclerosis. Thus, statin drugs could help prevent atherosclerosis by reducing inflammation, rather than by lowering cholesterol.[53] In this case, the much touted cholesterol-lowering action of these drugs could be largely an irrelevant side effect. A claim that it does not matter how statins work, as long as they do, is self-defeating. It means that researchers have investigated drugs for lowering cholesterol (a side effect) rather than concentrating on the actual mechanism. The likely result is that more effective treatments are overlooked.

The nature of corporate medicine is illustrated by the proposals for statin drugs. Dr. William Neal of West Virginia University has suggested that children ten or eleven years old have their cholesterol levels tested and managed with drugs. According to Neal, "Evidence suggests that treating children with elevated cholesterol reduces their risk of coronary heart disease later in life."[54] Such evidence is lacking for adults and is fundamentally absent for children. Studies to follow specific children, to determine their tendency to develop atherosclerosis late in life, would take decades, not to mention several generations of scientists. Furthermore, testing children at ten or eleven years old and treating them with statins would probably be unethical. Cholesterol is necessary for normal brain development. The statins would presumably be given throughout life, at unknowable risk to the children's future health. In addition, giving statins to a female who could later become pregnant may be harmful to the fetus. Some doctors, apparently half-jokingly, have suggested adding statins to the water supply. We find these wild claims for the indiscriminant use of statins shocking.

Nutrients

Fortunately, there are other ways to control blood lipid levels, which do not involve the risks and side effects associated with synthetic drugs. Since many of these are essential constituents of a healthy diet, they may offer side benefits, rather than dangerous side effects.

Niacin

One inexpensive nutrient that stands out as a cholesterol-lowering supplement is vitamin B_3 (niacin). High daily intakes of vitamin B_3 are more effective than currently available cholesterol-lowering drugs. In addition to these effects, niacin inhibits inflammation and protects the delicate linings of the arteries.[55] Niacin is an essential component of the diet and provides many health benefits.

There are several forms of vitamin B_3, including niacin (nicotinic acid), inositol hexanicotinate, and niacinamide (also called nicotinamide). They are mostly similar but niacin is preferable for preventing or treating heart disease. At high doses, niacin causes temporary skin flushing that starts in the face and travels down the body and limbs. Unless you want to cool yourself down, it is a good idea to wrap up well and conserve your body heat until the flushing subsides.

Some people consider a niacin flush to be a benefit or even a pleasure; it increases skin circulation and can relieve migraines. However, it can also be surprising or uncomfortable, especially if you are unaware that it might happen. Taking niacin with a meal can help minimize the supplement's skin-flushing effect. Another option is to choose no-flush or flush-free vitamin B_3 (inositol hexanicotinate), but it is worth noting that the mechanism that causes flushing may also help maintain the health of arterial walls. Importantly, the nicotinamide form does not have the same effects on the cardiovascular system as niacin, so they should not be used when the aim is to lower cholesterol.

Niacin supplements (1,000–2,000 milligrams taken three times a day) will lower "bad" LDL and lipoprotein(a) cholesterols. Lipoprotein(a) cholesterol is a form of LDL cholesterol. Furthermore, these intakes of niacin can increase the "good" HDL cholesterol,[56] restoring the blood lipid profile to one suggestive of

health.[57] Importantly, no current drug works as well as this vitamin. Niacin has also been shown to reduce the incidence of heart
attacks and to lower mortality in cardiac patients.[58] Niacin is one
of a range of B vitamins, which should be taken together. In addition to supplementing with niacin, a single B-100 tablet, taken
daily, should provide sufficient levels of the B-group vitamins.

At this point, you may be wondering why doctors advise
patients to take statin drugs, since niacin has been shown to be
effective. The real reason is probably that niacin is inexpensive and
easily available, and thus offers little potential for profit. However, your doctor may answer this question by referring to niacin's
side effects, such as skin flushing and the possibility of liver damage. We have already mentioned skin flushing. In regard to liver
damage, Dr. Abram Hoffer reported giving very high doses of
niacin to large numbers of patients for decades, without seeing a
single case of associated liver damage. It is worth noting that
Hoffer gave the niacin in combination with other B vitamins and
large doses of vitamin C, which would protect against free-radical
damage.

Use of high doses of niacin can increase liver enzymes, as can
many common over-the-counter drugs, such as aspirin or parac-
etamol (acetaminophen). The increase may not be problematic for
most healthy people; however, people who have liver-related illness should check with their doctor before taking high doses of
niacin. An informed family doctor should be able to monitor both
cholesterol levels and liver function, to put your mind at rest without raising undue concern over small changes in liver enzymes.

There are numerous other ways to lower cholesterol through
diet and nutrition, including food rich in phytosterols (such as
nuts, whole grains), which decrease its absorption from the intes-
tines, as well as garlic and foods high in soluble fiber. A niacin
supplement has the advantage that its action is direct, powerful,
and well established. For this reason, niacin should probably be
the first-line medication for people who want to lower their cholesterol levels.

Vitamin E

Vitamin E is often recommended for heart disease. There are many forms of vitamin E, such as the tocotrienols and the more commonly known tocopherols. At high intakes (1,000 IU or more daily), mixed natural tocopherols may help prevent and treat cardiovascular disease. The tocotrienols also have some particularly interesting properties and may reverse atherosclerosis, as well as improving blood cholesterol levels.[59] Although they are not the common form of vitamin E (i.e. tocopherols), tocotrienols are available as supplements. Try to find natural supplements that contain mainly tocotrienols, as the common tocopherol form may inhibit absorption when taken at the same time. Aim to supplement with at least 100 milligrams of mixed natural tocotrienols a day. Natural forms of vitamin E are absorbed and utilized better than synthetic forms, which should be avoided.

Vitamin C

At high blood levels, vitamin C will also improve blood cholesterol levels[60] and has been proposed as a treatment for high blood cholesterol and hypercholesterolemia.[61] Some studies in healthy young patients suggest that vitamin C lowers blood cholesterol, though the reports are not consistent.[62] The vitamin's action appears to depend on the size of the intake and current health condition of the person who takes it.

In people with existing atherosclerosis, a daily 1-gram dose of vitamin C may even raise blood cholesterol. This could be because the vitamin removes cholesterol from the arterial walls and plaques into the blood, thereby increasing the blood levels.[63] Despite this increase, the risk of heart attack would diminish. The important point is what happens in the artery wall; cholesterol in the blood is a side issue.[64] In addition to lowering cholesterol levels, vitamin C prevents it from oxidizing and causing harm.

Revising the "cholesterol is bad" theory to "oxidized cholesterol is bad" suggests a way of preventing heart disease and has the advantage of relating cholesterol to free-radical damage and inflammation within the arterial wall. On the other hand, it does not explain why the oxidized cholesterol would build up in the arterial wall specifically, rather than in other tissues. If cholesterol oxidation could be prevented, the risk of atherosclerosis might vanish. A suitable antioxidant should ideally be a normal, safe part of the diet. In this modified approach, provided there are sufficient antioxidants, high blood cholesterol may not lead to atherosclerosis.

To be effective in preventing atherosclerosis, the intake of vitamin C should be at least 1,000 milligrams, taken three or four times a day (a total of about 4 grams a day). Some people may require more and a few may need less, but this regimen represents the smallest intake that is likely to be effective.

DIETARY FATS

It is possible to make dietary changes that will improve your blood lipid levels with a higher degree of safety than using drugs. This section is mainly about dietary fats, however, we should also point out that reducing your intake of carbohydrates, particularly the sugar fructose, will lower your blood cholesterol. Fructose is also known as fruit sugar, it is found in table sugar (sucrose) and, as the name suggests, in high-fructose corn syrup (HFCS). Some incorrectly consider fruit sugar healthy, but fructose is harmful—it will both raise and disrupt your cholesterol levels. Those who subscribe to the cholesterol theory would do well to stop criticizing saturated fat in the diet and concentrate on this sugar.

People are often urged to reduce their intake of fat, but this advice is an extreme oversimplification. Some fats lower the risk of heart disease, while others increase it. Researchers have even suggested the creation of fat-enriched foods, which contain fish oils, to reduce the risk of heart disease.[65] Clearly, there is more to reducing your risk of heart disease than just cutting back your fat intake.

The saturated fats in the diet are often said to be harmful, but are largely safe. Strangely, the medical establishment has sometimes recommended replacing safe fats in the diet with potentially harmful alternatives. For many years, people have been advised to avoid saturated fat and to replace it with polyunsaturated oils. We are told to eat margarine rather than butter; supposedly, the polyunsaturated fat in margarine will reduce our risk of heart disease, whereas the saturated fat in butter is branded as harmful. In order to appreciate the relevance of such claims and, more importantly, their limitations, we need to understand the difference between these types of fat.

Types of Fat

Both oils and fats are lipids, but oils are liquid at room temperature, whereas fats are solid. Chemically, both fats and oils contain fatty acids, which are chains of carbon and hydrogen atoms, ending in an acidic chemical group. Saturated fats are made up of fatty acids that contain a maximum number of hydrogen atoms; their name reflects the fact that they are "saturated" with hydrogen atoms.

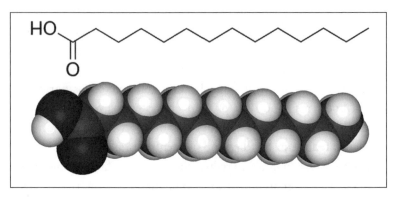

SATURATED FAT CONTAINS SINGLE BONDS, IN A STRAIGHT CHAIN, WITH AN (OOH) ACID GROUP AT THE END.

An unsaturated fat contains at least one double bond between two of its carbon atoms. Two hydrogen atoms are removed to create the extra bond between the carbon atoms, so unsaturated fat has fewer hydrogen atoms.

Polyunsaturated fats contain more than one double bond, and they are bent, or kinked, which prevents them from being arranging into a solid array. So, polyunsaturated oils are typically liquid, whereas saturated fat is solid. Correspondingly, vegetable cooking oils are often unsaturated, whereas butter is saturated.

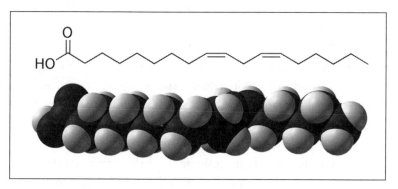

UNSATURATED FAT CONTAINS DOUBLE BONDS, CAUSING THE CHAIN TO KINK.

Rancidity

Typically, oils and fats, such as butter, have a high affinity for oxygen. If oils are left in contact with air, most will turn rancid. The first scientist to investigate this phenomenon was Nicolas de Saussure, a Swiss pioneer of plant physiology. Saussure discovered that plants generate sugar from carbon dioxide and water during photosynthesis. In about 1820, he observed that a layer of walnut oil on water absorbed three times its own volume of air in eight months. The reaction then progressed quickly, such that, in only ten days, the oil absorbed sixty times its own volume. Over the next three months, the uptake slowed, until about 145 times the volume of the oil was absorbed.

The reaction of oils with oxygen has been considered sufficiently important to be given its own name: peroxidation. Peroxidation starts when hydrogen atoms are removed from the carbon backbone of a fatty acid. Saturated fats are more resistant than polyunsaturated fats, which contain reactive double bonds. Fish oil supplements, containing large amounts of polyunsaturated fatty acids, are particularly prone to such oxidation. For this reason, once opened, fish oil supplements should be kept refrigerated, in closed containers, away from light. Unless these supplements are stored properly, their nutritional value will quickly decline. Fish oil supplements often contain an antioxidant, such as vitamin E, to help prevent peroxidation and maintain freshness.

That fats become rancid is not just a concern when it comes to our food. Each human cell has a lipid membrane—a thin layer of fat—that is subject to oxidative damage in a similar manner. The bag-like membrane is essential to contain the cellular contents. Since the membrane forms the cell's outside surface, it is in contact with oxygen and other chemicals in its surroundings. Fortunately, vitamin E and other fat-soluble antioxidants help prevent oxidation of cell membranes and of other fats and oils in the body. If these antioxidant defenses fail, damaging free radicals are formed. A single oxidized fat molecule becomes a free radical, starting a chain reaction that can attack and damage the cells' structure or biochemistry.

It is sensible to avoid eating foods containing oxidized or rancid fats. Feeding large amounts of oxidized fat to animals such as rabbits and rats leads to severe problems, including heart damage and fatty liver.[66] However, the toxicity is relatively low.[67] Animals can often metabolize these fats and minimize their damaging effects; their guts are able to detoxify many peroxides as they are being absorbed.[68] For humans, eating oxidized fat is unwise, but the saturated fats in fresh butter are relatively safe.

Saturated Fat

Saturated fats, such as butter and lard, are described by corporate medicine as a risk factor for heart disease. Once again, however, the evidence is indirect and rather flimsy. The late Dr. Robert Atkins famously recommended a weight loss diet that was high in saturated fat and low in carbohydrates. The Atkins Diet was popular, though a source of great controversy.[69] Since a high-fat diet was thought to be a cause of heart disease, such a diet should, in theory, be deadly. Atkins was a cardiologist turned orthomolecular physician and did not believe a high-fat diet caused heart attacks. Despite this, he was criticized for promoting a diet that would endanger people's lives by giving them heart disease. Indeed, it was wrongly suggested that even studies on the danger of this diet might be less than ethical because of the perceived danger.[69] However, failing to investigate the diet would put prejudice above science.

The conventional view was that Atkins' suggestions ran contrary to the laws of physics: a person could only lose weight by taking in less energy, in other words, by eating fewer calories. Atkins seemed to be saying people could eat as much as they liked and still lose weight.[70] His real argument—that people who eat fat and protein feel full for longer and therefore eat less—was misunderstood. It did not occur to the medical establishment that their own recommendations for a high carbohydrate, low-fat diet would make people hungry, fat, and leave them at high risk of heart attack.

Atkin's low-carbohydrate diet proved surprisingly effective for weight loss. At the time it was introduced, popular diets involved cutting calories and reducing fat intake, resulting in a restricted diet, high in carbohydrates. The Atkins approach was often found to produce superior weight loss to such diets.[71] The results of these trials were reproducible, as was the skepticism with which they were received.[72] Low carbohydrate fad diets were described as nutritional nonsense, and they were presumed guilty unless "proven" otherwise.[73]

Besides being good for losing weight, the Atkins Diet appears to lower risk factors for heart disease,[74] including the newer risk factors.[75] Eating fat seems to provide a healthier balance of blood lipid levels. Indeed, lipid-lowering drugs may be unnecessary for many patients, as reducing carbohydrate intake can work just as well.[76] Corporate medicine contends that this just should not happen—but it does.

Low-carbohydrate diets are intrinsically healthy. Restricting car-

THE OFFICIAL FOOD PYRAMID

To help people select healthy food, organizations such as the U.S. Department of Agriculture (USDA) have proposed a food pyramid. Unfortunately, their pyramid recommends eating foods containing large amounts of carbohydrate. The main exception is sweets or candies, which are correctly placed at the peak of the pyramid, indicating the lowest recommended intake. We include the USDA food pyramid diagram from 1992 for illustration.

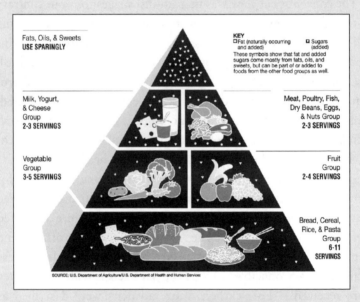

FOOD PYRAMID (1992)

Recent USDA guidelines from 2005 are overloaded with sugar.[77] They recommend consuming "two cups of fruit and 2.5 cups of vegetables per day." Eating plenty of vegetables is fine, but many common fruits, such as apples and bananas, contain relatively large amounts of available sugar. The official suggestion to mix colors of fruit and vegetables is a sensible way of obtaining a range of phytonutrients but, again, this needs to be balanced against the quantities of sugar in some fruit.

The USDA guidelines also recommend six or more ounces of grains each day, such as wheat or rice, at least half of which are whole grain. Even whole-grain wheat consists of about 73 percent carbohydrate, with 12 percent fiber. White flour is about 74 percent carbohydrate, with only 3 percent fiber. Grains are laden with starch and sugar, although whole grains release their sugars more slowly than milled grains do. For this reason, whole grain is often described as having a low glycemic index (GI), which relates to how quickly the sugars are made available to the body.

For dairy, the recommended intake is 3 cups of low-fat or fat-free milk each day. While low-fat and fat-free milk has its fat removed, it still contains relatively large amounts of the sugar lactose. Lactose is not particularly sweet, so many people do not realize that cow's milk contains about the same amount of sugar as a cola drink. Each liter of milk contains almost 50 grams of lactose, equivalent to 10 teaspoons of sugar. Because dietary guidelines call for a reduced intake of saturated fat, cholesterol, and trans-fat, presumably any milk included in the diet should be skimmed, which many people think is healthy and slimming; however, skimmed milk contains less fat and more sugar than full cream milk.

What we need to remember is that, for humans, agriculture is a recent technology. Only for the last 10,000 years have we farmed grains such as wheat and rice. In evolutionary terms, this period is barely the blink of an eye. For most of human existence, hunter-gatherers appear to have lived on a diet of vegetables, with what little added meat or fish they could catch.[78] This means we evolved eating a low-carbohydrate diet.

The USDA food pyramid recommends eating more of the foods at the base and less of those at the top. Compared with the official version, a more appropriate pyramid would recommend large amounts of vegetables, as they typically contain nutrients, dietary fiber, and little available sugar. Fish would also be at the base, provided it was not contaminated with pollutants, such as mercury; it is high in protein and contains beneficial oils. Saturated fat and cholesterol would be given the benefit of the doubt and meat would be placed in the middle. Carbohydrates and sugar-rich foods, including many fruits, would be up near the peak, as they are typically less healthy. Many so-called healthy drinks, such as fruit juice, would be included with the discouraged foods at the top of the pyramid, alongside sugar and prepared foods containing high-fructose corn syrup. Most people agree that trans-fats are harmful, so they should be excluded.

bohydrates reduces body fat and lowers blood insulin.[79] However, corporate medicine's prejudice against fat is such that a low-fat, high-carbohydrate diet is recommended, even for diabetics. This ignores the apparent irrationality of increasing carbohydrate (i.e. sugar) intake to manage a disease in which the body cannot process and control sugar. Even worse, in diabetic foods, such as chocolate, the sweetener used is often fructose—a particularly dangerous sugar. Lowering the carbohydrate intake of diabetics is a rational therapeutic approach.[80,81] A suitable low-carbohydrate diet can reverse type 2 diabetes in weeks and can reduce the dose of insulin for people with type 1 diabetes.

Even based on the accepted risk factors, the argument that a diet high in saturated fat and low in carbohydrates will increase blood cholesterol and thus cause heart disease is incorrect. The real problem with low-carbohydrate diets is not that they increase heart-disease risk, but that they can cause nutritional deficiencies, due to a decreased dietary intake of vitamins, minerals, and phytochemicals.[82] The Atkins Diet is beneficial for weight loss, but it is too extreme for good health. The more recently popular Paleolithic (paleo or primal) diets include more vegetables, while keeping carbohydrate intake low.

Trans-Fats

As the theory that high-fat diets were responsible for heart disease took hold back in the 1950s, the myth that margarine's hydrogenated oils and trans-fats were healthier than butter became popular. Trans-fats are formed when vegetable oil is hydrogenated, during the manufacture of margarine. Partial hydrogenation involves heating liquid vegetable oils in the presence of metal catalysts and hydrogen. This process causes some of the fatty acid's molecules to straighten, making it easier for the molecules to attract each other. The resulting trans-fat is typically solid at room temperature. The more naturally occurring unsaturated cis-fatty acids have a more curved shape, so they do not combine as easily and typically remain liquid at room temperature.

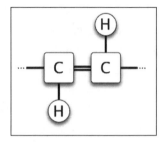

TRANS-FAT

We agree with the official recommendations that intake of trans-fatty acids should be kept as low as possible, while consuming a nutritionally adequate diet. Trans-fatty acids are not essential to human health and provide no known benefit.[83] Trans-fats have more adverse effects on blood lipid levels than saturated fats.[84] These harmful fats are used to increase the shelf life and flavor stability of processed food. Margarine and vegetable shortenings are sources of trans-fat in the diet.

Trans-fats are used by the food industry instead of solid fats and liquid oils from natural sources. This replacement has been greatest in the realm of fast food. A cracker that remains crisp, despite being left on the shelf for months, is a consequence of the use of trans-fat. Snack food, baked goods, and processed foods often contain high levels of trans-fat.

Commercial production of partially hydrogenated fats began in the early twentieth century and increased steadily until about the 1960s. Since then, processed vegetable fats have tended to displace animal fats in Western diets. The initial motivation was to lower costs, but companies soon began to claim health benefits for margarine as a replacement for butter. This specious hype continues to this day.

The strange health claims for margarine were supported by corporate medicine's acceptance that saturated fat and cholesterol in the diet were causes of heart disease. While soft margarine manufacturers have now reduced their use of trans-fats, the average consumption did not change greatly from the 1960s to the start of the new century, because of increased use in commercial products and fast foods.[85] Not surprisingly, margarine and food producers suggest that trans-fats occur naturally in dairy products, meat, and poultry. Only a strict vegan diet might contain no trans-fats, or trace levels. However, there is suggestive evidence that not all trans-fats are equally damaging to health. Some naturally occurring fats may have a configuration similar to trans-fats, but could be safe or even beneficial.[86] Natural and synthetic trans-fats are different substances.

As the fable that cholesterol and saturated fat causes heart disease became more widely accepted, butter began to be replaced with artificial spreads that were promoted as healthy and of particular benefit to those with heart disease. People who hoped to minimize their risk of heart attack were misguided into substituting harmful margarines for the butter in their diets. In 1997, a group of doctors and scientists from Harvard and other Boston institutions followed up the Nurses' Health Study, originally published by Walter Willett and colleagues in *The Lancet*.[87] The follow-up collected data from 80,082 nurses, for a period of fourteen years, and documented 939 cases of heart attack.[88] The authors suggested that a 5 percent increase in saturated fat raised the risk of coronary disease by 17 percent, when compared with carbohydrates. However, an increase of only 2 percent in trans-fat intake produced a 93 percent greater risk than carbohydrates.

The replacement of saturated fat by trans-fat is increasingly realized to be a grave error. The widespread publicity campaigns against butter and other saturated fats occurred at a time of increased consumption of trans-fats. Over a period spanning several decades, health concerns were raised about trans-fats in the diet and the associated risk of heart disease.[89] Epidemiological studies linked trans-fats to increased risk of coronary heart disease. In 1994, it was estimated that trans-fats might be responsible for 30,000 premature coronary heart disease deaths each year in the U.S.[90] As might be expected, the food industry responded that the evidence was not sufficient to justify taking action. They made the claim, common to so many students' essays, that further research was needed.[91] A decade later, however, it was accepted that trans-fats were more harmful than saturated fats.

There is no safe level of artificial trans-fat intake. Data on the harmful effects of trans-fats continue to accumulate and researchers have suggested that thousands of lives might be saved by limiting people's intake of trans-fats.[92] The *British Medical Journal* has recently called for them to be removed from the food supply.[93] New U.S. Food and Drug Administration (FDA) guidelines mean that trans-fat has a partial listing on food labels in the United States. The addition of trans-fats is even banned from some supermarkets and restaurants. Despite this, the evidence is that trans-fat is another risk factor for heart disease, rather than a direct cause.

EATING FAT TO STAY THIN

Fat was not always condemned: those of us who were raised in the '50s and '60s remember our mothers warning us against sweet candies or starchy potatoes, because "they will make you fat." The more recent fashion for low-fat diets goes against this common-sense approach. Cholesterol has been given an evil reputation and it is about time it was rehabilitated. In itself, saturated fat in the diet does not appear to be harmful.

Dr. Atkins' book was certainly not the first to suggest a low-carbohydrate diet. William Banting described a similar diet in his 1865 *Letter on Corpulence*.[94] This followed an even earlier book called *The Physiology of Taste,* written by Jean Anthelme Brillat-Savarin in 1825.[95] Brillat-Savarin believed that sugar, white flour, and starchy vegetables caused obesity. To stay slim, he suggested

Fat Fallacies

Cholesterol and saturated fat should be removed from the diet?
This book should leave little doubt that cholesterol is essential to health and its presence in the diet is harmless. Moreover, saturated fat in the diet is not a cause of heart disease or stroke. Saturated fat becomes unhealthy if it is oxidized; for example, by burning during cooking or if rancid butter is eaten.

Trans-fatty acids in the diet are as dangerous as saturated fat?
Since there is little harm from typical saturated fats, this statement is incorrect. However, trans-fats are dangerous and should be avoided, as they can promote inflammation in the arteries.

Margarine is healthier than butter.
Margarine was initially introduced to the poor and lower classes as an inexpensive substitute for butter. Its popularity increased during the First World War and again during the Second World War, when dairy products became scarce. More recently, the margarine lobby has attempted to market margarine as a "health food."

Margarines can include a variety of animal or vegetable fats, in an emulsion of 80 percent fat and 20 percent water, together with various coloring agents and additives. Although margarines have often contained dangerous hydrogenated and trans-fats, the health benefits claimed by manufacturers generally depend on their lower cholesterol or saturated fat content compared with butter. Unless you are a strict vegetarian or vegan, we suggest that butter is preferable and is a more healthy food.

Unsaturated vegetable oil is healthy?
Saturated vegetable oils tend to be solid at room temperature and have a short storage time and shelf life. Unsaturated oils are generally liquid at room temperature. There seems to be a limited sort of reasoning along the lines that thin liquid oils will not clog up arteries as much as thick fats. However, many vegetable cooking oils degrade and oxidize, forming toxins at high temperatures.

Olive, hemp, and macadamia oils are examples of vegetable oils that contain high proportions of monounsaturated oils, as well as natural antioxidants. Fish and krill oils are polyunsaturated oils that are considered healthy, provided they are of supplement grade and are kept refrigerated once opened. More generally, polyunsaturated food oils, such as canola cooking oil, are best avoided.

Coconut oil is unhealthy
This is another myth. Despite its name, coconut oil is a healthy, largely saturated fat and is solid at room temperature. It is resistant to oxidation and has a long shelf life, even at room temperature, without going rancid. Coconut oil is stable at high temperatures and makes an excellent cooking oil. It has a high proportion of short chain molecules, making it particularly easy to digest. Some hair care and skin care products also contain coconut oil.

Rather than being a source of allegedly harmful saturated fats, coconut oil offers numerous health benefits. The list is long and includes improved digestion, increased immunity, enhanced metabolism, stress relief, and weight loss. There are some claims that coconut oil can prevent kidney problems and cancer, as well as aiding dental care. This saturated fat has also been suggested as a preventative for diabetes, high blood pressure, and cardiovascular diseases.

Rules of Thumb

- Avoid so-called "healthy" margarine and trans-fats.
- Enjoy butter.
- Replace vegetable cooking oils with olive/coconut oil.
- Coconut oil is an excellent food and cooking aid.
- Saturated fat is not the enemy.
- Trans-fat is bad.
- Cholesterol is good.
- Supplement your diet with omega-3 fish oil.

a protein-rich, low-carbohydrate diet. Brillat-Savarin explained that carnivorous animals, such as wolves, jackals, birds of prey, and crows, never grow fat. Herbivores living on a vegetable diet also stay quite slim, until old age renders them inactive. However, vegetarian animals fatten quickly if they are fed a diet of potatoes, grain or flour. Brillat-Savarin's famous quote is: "Tell me what you eat and I'll tell you what you are."

A low-carbohydrate diet is less harmful than the low-fat diets recommended by government agencies. Over the last 30–40 years, the introduction of these low-fat guidelines has coincided with epidemics of obesity, type 2 diabetes, and other health problems. The low-fat "healthy option" processed foods found in supermarkets are often loaded with sugar, high-fructose corn syrup, salt, and additives. In effect, the authorities have been pushing us to eat junk food that will make us fat and give us heart disease.

Confusion arising from population studies has maintained the belief that saturated fat causes heart disease. More recently, recommendations to replace saturated fat with hydrogenated vegetable oils and trans-fats are seen to have been an error. The evidence for the actions of both fat and cholesterol in the development of coronary heart disease indicates that they are minor risk factors and are not the primary cause of the disease.

IMPORTANT POINTS

- Cholesterol in the normal diet does not lead to high blood cholesterol.

- High blood cholesterol is a failure of the body's internal controls.

- Cholesterol does not cause heart disease.

- Official dietary recommendations have been consistently wrong.

- Low-fat diets are harmful.

CHAPTER 5

SWEET BUT DEADLY

"If only a small fraction of what is already known about the effects of sugar were to be revealed in relation to any other material used as a food additive, that material would promptly be banned."

—JOHN YUDKIN

Sugar makes people fat and unhealthy—most people know this. What they may not realize is that many foods that are recommended by the U.S. Department of Agriculture—such as those that form the base of the food pyramid—contain large quantities of starch and sugar. Furthermore, many "healthy" low-fat supermarket foods contain excessive sugar, as do soft drinks and fruit juices. These sugar-laden foods are the cause of the modern obesity epidemic. Contrary to popular belief, fat-free foods are far from healthy.

There is more reason to reduce sugar in the diet than to reduce cholesterol. Dr. John Yudkin, an eminent professor of physiology at the University of London, publicized the involvement of sugar in heart disease in his acclaimed book *Pure, White and Deadly*.[1] He described the relationship between sugar intake and rates of coronary heart disease. Furthermore, atherosclerosis, heart disease, and stroke are well-known complications for diabetics, who suffer from increased blood glucose levels.

In arterial plaques, molecules in the blood vessel wall are cross-linked by glucose, a process known as glycation. This process is involved in the development of high blood pressure and the aging of arteries. As a result of glycation, glucose acts as a bridge between collagen and other molecules in blood vessel walls, making the walls stiffer. The reduced elasticity means that normal expansion of the blood vessels requires higher blood pressures. Glucose and other sugars are thus a noteworthy feature in arteriosclerosis, which is the aging and hardening of arteries. As the arteries stiffen, stress on the arterial walls increases, especially in areas of high curvature and fast blood flow, such as the aortic arch (where the main artery leaves the heart and then bends sharply) and the coronary vessels that are implicated in heart attacks.

Obesity reflects a failure of the body's internal controls. Contrary to popular opinion, people rarely become obese just because they are lazy or greedy. They eat more because the natural mechanisms that should tell them when they have eaten enough have stopped working properly. As a result, they continue to feel hungry, so they keep on eating. Few people actually want to get fat—they just can't help themselves. Overeating by a few mouthfuls a day can make the difference between being fat or skinny. People who blame others for being overweight would do well to remember that, over time, just a slight difference in energy intake can cause a large change in body fat.

In some ways, our bodies and particularly our minds are not well equipped to cope with modern excesses. Long ago, humans evolved in an environment quite different from today's fast-food culture. Our ancestors could not pop down to the local take-out place if they were hungry. They had to eat food when they could, building up fat reserves in times of plenty against the near-certainty of famine in the future. When food became scarce, individuals with the ability to eat a lot and store food as fat gained a survival advantage. They passed this advantage on to us, their descendants. Unfortunately, in modern Western societies, with our constant food supplies, there is nothing to stop people from eating just a little too much each day until we become massively overweight, suffer chronic disease, and die.

Some of the things we eat, especially sugars, confuse the body's controls. This can lead to a condition with a variety of names, such as insulin resistance, metabolic syndrome, type 2 diabetes, and syndrome X. These terms are associated with obesity and heart disease. People with metabolic syndrome tend to put on weight, especially around the waist. They may find it hard to lose the weight even if they try to control their eating and get more exercise. Such people may find that diet and exercise will take off a few pounds, but the fat around their middle does not budge. The conventional low-fat and calorie-counting diets they are urged to follow simply do not work for any length of time.

Ironically, governments and industry have spent billions advising us to eat the same high-carbohydrate, low-fat foods that cause the problem. Furthermore, mainstream dieticians seem to agree: the American Dietetic Association says we should search our supermarkets for "fruits and vegetables from the produce aisles, whole grains from the bakery, low-fat milk products from the dairy case, and lean proteins from the meat/fish/poultry department." Three of these categories (fruit, grains, and low-fat milk products) are likely to be high in sugar. The British Dietetic Association also recommends that people "choose lower-fat foods, e.g., lean meat and lower-fat dairy products." Supporters of more rational diets—which could enable people to lose weight, prevent metabolic syndrome, and avoid heart attacks—are kept to the fringes of nutrition or even derided as credulous and naïve.

OVERWEIGHT

Lack of exercise plays a part in our expanding waistlines. From a young age, we are getting less exercise than our parents did. In 1969, four in ten U.S. children walked to school; by 2001, the number had fallen to just over one in ten.[2] Exercise increases muscle mass, raises the metabolism, and counters type 2 diabetes.

The benefits of exercise are not simply about burning calories, however. An adult would need to walk about 20 miles to get rid of the calories in a single Big Mac meal. Lack of exercise does not explain the epidemic of obesity; thin people are couch potatoes, too.

Sadly, it is not just adults who are piling on the weight: babies less than six months old are becoming fat.[3] Lack of exercise does not explain obese babies. The two most plausible explanations relate to baby food and to what mothers eat, during or before pregnancy and while breastfeeding. One possible cause is increased consumption of monosodium glutamate (MSG) and related flavor enhancers.[4] A second candidate is over-consumption of sugar, which can result in obesity and heart disease.

A healthy body can regulate its own weight by assessing the food eaten against the energy expended. This is a delicate balance. Eating a mere 100 calories or so extra each day for a year will add about ten pounds to your weight. However, it is extremely difficult to eat a few grams less each day in order to lose that excess fat. Our conscious eating controls are simply not that precise.

If you are overweight, it may not be through gluttony, lack of willpower, or motivation. You could be living an active life and trying hard to control your eating. The cause may be *what* you are eating, rather than the amount. Some foodstuffs, like MSG and sugar, can lead you to feel hungrier and trick you into overeating instead of satisfying your appetite. Some additives and sweeteners affect your body's internal controls, which would normally tell you when to stop eating. People who want to retain a trim figure or to slim down might do well to avoid MSG, which is often hidden behind obscure labeling in processed foods. However, lowering your sugar intake is a more reliable route to weight loss.

The usual criticism of sugars is that they provide empty calories. This means they supply energy, but no vitamins or other nutrients. However, this is an oversimplification. Glucose provides the body with pure energy, without any other nutrition. More dis-

turbingly, other sugars are not necessarily just empty calories—
they can be poisons.

FATTENING CARBOHYDRATES

Humans, other animals, and plants all need glucose. Plants manufacture glucose from carbon dioxide and water during photosynthesis, the main provider of energy for life on earth. They use it to
make a vital structural component, cellulose, which consists of
long chains of glucose molecules linked together by chemical
bonds. Cellulose forms much of the dietary fiber in fruit and vegetables, but humans and other mammals cannot digest it. Some
bacteria are able to break down the bonds in cellulose, and animals such as cows have these bacteria in their guts, allowing them
to digest cellulose-rich grasses.

Like cellulose, starch is made from chains of glucose, but the
molecules are not linked together in the same way. Rather than
forming long fibers, the glucose molecules in starch are more
branched and form granules. In plants, starch is the major energy
store and forms the bulk of many vegetables, including potatoes,
carrots, turnips, peas, and sweet corn (maize). Animals have
enzymes to break down starch and use it as a source of glucose.
Unlike plants, however, we store our excess energy as fat.

Disregarding added sugars, starch is usually the main carbohydrate in the diet. Most staples of the modern diet, such as bread,
rice, potatoes, noodles, and porridge, consist of starchy foods. As
soon as starch is chewed in the mouth, it begins to break down.
An enzyme called amylase in saliva starts splitting the starch into
glucose, even before it reaches the stomach. Because of this breakdown, a starch-rich baked potato can cause a rapid increase in
blood sugar. The glycemic index (GI) is a measure of how quickly a food is converted to glucose in the blood. A baked potato has
a high GI (about 85), whereas a typical chocolate candy, such as
a Mars bar, has a lower GI (only 65). Even table sugar has a GI
of only about 61, which is a medium level compared to a potato.

It seems strange that a food that is normally considered healthy, such as a baked potato, can provide a faster increase in blood sugar than eating table sugar (sucrose) itself. The difference is in the type of sugar.

When doctors talk about blood sugar, they are usually referring to glucose. A baked potato is mostly starch and water; when digested, it generates a glucose solution that is rapidly absorbed. Glucose is not particularly sweet to the taste—a baked potato does not taste sweet, even though it releases glucose in the mouth. By contrast, table sugar (sucrose) consists of glucose molecules linked to another sugar, fructose, and is about 25 percent sweeter than glucose.

When you eat foods containing sucrose, the sugar gets split into its components, glucose and fructose. The glucose can go straight into the blood, but the fructose is stored in the liver. Consequently, table sugar (medium GI) does not increase blood glucose as much as a baked potato (high GI). Almost half the sucrose goes into the liver, lowering the impact on the blood levels. As sugars go, however, glucose is relatively safe, so despite its high GI, a baked potato is healthier than a high-fructose cola drink.

THE SUGAR THAT ROTS YOUR TEETH

In the past, dentists recommended that people eat apples rather than candy, reasoning that a candy bar contains table sugar, which rots your teeth and causes cavities. These days, dentists are less keen on apples, which contain high levels of sugar as well as acids that cause dental erosion. Dried apples are almost 60 percent carbohydrate. Apple juice contains a lot of sugar, of which about half is fructose and the rest a mixture of glucose and sucrose.[5] The amounts vary with the variety of apple.[6]

Nevertheless, the type of sugar in apples is better for your teeth than that in candies. An apple's combination of fructose along with lesser quantities of glucose and sucrose is less damaging to teeth than the high levels of sucrose in candies. In addition, the sugars in whole apples are less readily available, because they are enclosed within cellulose cell walls.

A dentist who recommends choosing an apple rather than a candy bar is trying to protect your teeth by lowering your intake of sucrose. Bacteria on teeth can turn table sugar into lactic acid, which dissolves enamel, creating cavities. Table sugar plays a particular and central role in rotting teeth, though this fact is not always fully explained by dentists. The main bacterium of interest is called *Streptococcus mutans*. This bug manufactures lactic acid from many sugars, including glucose, fructose, and even lactose (the sugar found in milk). An important distinction, however, is that *S. mutans* uses sucrose to form a kind of glue, with which it sticks itself to the tooth enamel, helping to form plaque. This is what leads to common table sugar being a specific cause of tooth decay and gum disease. Sucrose is a particularly poor choice of sugar if you wish to maintain good dental health.

Dentists often encourage the use of fluoride, a potent toxin, for prevention of dental caries. In 2006, the American Association of Poison Control Centers reported over 21,000 exposures involving fluoride toothpaste.[7] Most of these incidents concerned young children. The fluoride that is added to drinking water is an industrial waste product of the fertilizer industry. While most people are concerned about removing pollutants from the water supply, toxic fluoride is promoted. Fluoridation would be unnecessary if people switched from using table sugar to using glucose as a sweetener, which could help prevent many cavities from developing in the first place. It would also help protect against heart disease, as the fructose in table sugar is a strong candidate for being a food that destroys the cardiovascular system.

PURE, WHITE, AND DEADLY

David Kritchevsky, a biochemist who was still publishing until he died in 2006 at the age of eighty-six, was one of the first scientists to study the link between cholesterol and cardiovascular risk. He pointed out that rabbits fed a diet high in sugar and saturated fat can suffer a form of atherosclerosis, even when the diet contains no cholesterol. Furthermore, he claimed, addition of saturated fat to laboratory chow (food pellets) does not cause atherosclerosis and cardiovascular disease. His work suggests that, in animals, sugar or starch—rather than saturated fat—is responsible.[8]

Fructose is the primary sugar that damages your heart. In 1972, John Yudkin described the relationship between sugar and cardiovascular disease.[9] The idea that too much sugar is harmful brought Yudkin into conflict with powerful lobbies, but he was never afraid to question established dogma.[10] Naturally, corporate medicine ignored the issue. After all, there was too great an investment in the belief that cholesterol was the primary culprit in heart disease—changing tack would have meant dismantling research teams, finding new funding, and starting again from scratch. Food manufacturers similarly had large investments in sugar. The idea that the sugar in your diet was more harmful than saturated fat was too inconvenient to be taken seriously.

Fructose is more damaging than glucose, lactose (milk sugar), or sorbitol (a sugar alcohol). Feeding fructose to baboons increases their cholesterol levels and damages their arteries, and similar arterial inflammation is observed in monkeys.[11] Mice also get a form of atherosclerosis when fed fructose.[12] In these animal models, the atherosclerosis generated following consumption of fructose does not depend on increased blood cholesterol.[13] So, even if you believe the cholesterol theory, you should remove fructose from your diet, rather than cholesterol. If you eat common table sugar (sucrose) you are risking atherosclerosis, obesity, and increased insulin resistance.[14] Excess fructose is not merely extra calories; it acts as a poison, producing numerous health problems.

HEART DISEASE STARTS IN CHILDHOOD

Generally, we think of heart disease as something that happens to older people. Sadly, however, the early stages of atherosclerosis and related conditions, such as adult-onset diabetes, are increasingly found in children. Diabetes can lead to serious complications, including heart disease, stroke, loss of limbs, and blindness. In healthy people, blood sugar levels are controlled by the hormone insulin. For people with type 1 diabetes, insulin is absent—the body is unable to make it or can only produce it in small quantities. Type 2 diabetes is less drastic: either the body does not make enough insulin or the cells cannot respond to the insulin signal to convert glucose to energy. Cells that are less able to respond to the hormone are called insulin resistant.

Type 2 diabetes is often referred to as late or adult-onset diabetes. This description separates it from type 1 diabetes, which often starts during childhood. These days, however, "late" onset diabetes is found in more and more children; this increase is associated with obesity. Children are getting fat and developing adult-onset diabetes. In children, metabolic syndrome leads to premature atherosclerosis and increases the risk that they may suffer a heart attack or stroke relatively early in life.[15] Chronic illness that is normally associated with aging is starting to afflict young people. The cause of diabetic illness in children appears to be an increase in their intake of sugars, particularly fructose. The same effect occurs in animals. When hamsters are given a high-fructose diet, they develop metabolic syndrome rather quickly. For this reason, hamsters fed fructose are used as an experimental model for metabolic syndrome and type 2 diabetes.

Fructose is a cause of high blood pressure. It appears to increase the oxidation of cholesterol in damaged arterial walls, which leads to atherosclerosis.[16] Like glucose, fructose can cause cross-linking of proteins and other large molecules, but it does so more quickly. In arterial walls, cross-linking by fructose hardens the arteries, generating high blood pressure and premature aging. During cooking, fructose is often used to create an appealing brown color on foods, such as the surface of cakes. This browning occurs because fructose is easily oxidized and degraded by heat. Unfortunately, the same effect can occur in the body, where oxidation is less attractive: the browning of the surface in cooked cakes is more appealing than wrinkles in human skin.

The idea that fructose is "healthy" may have arisen because it does not lead to an immediate increase in blood sugar.[17] However, in the long term, it is far more harmful than glucose. Essentially, when we eat fructose, it is transferred to the liver, where it is converted into fat and increases "bad" LDL cholesterol in the blood. Since sucrose molecules consist of glucose linked to fructose, eating sucrose is similarly harmful, though only half as bad as if we ate pure fructose. The historical choice of sucrose as our main dietary sugar was unfortunate.

Another reason fructose may have been considered more healthy than other sugars is because it is often described as "fruit sugar" and associated with common fruit, which is seen as natural and can even be organic. Do not be fooled by this marketing hype. When eaten, whole fruit releases relatively small amounts of fructose over time; fruits also contain vitamins, fiber and other nutrients, so they do not present an overall health risk. By comparison, fruit juice contains troubling levels of available fructose, because the fibrous cell walls that enclose the sugar in the whole fruit have been smashed up by the juicer. The sugar in juice goes straight into your system, rather than being slowly absorbed and allowing your metabolism time to adapt. For this reason, fruit juice should be avoided; it may sound contrarian but juice is not the same as whole fruit and may contain similar sugar levels to fizzy soda.

Encouraging our children to drink soda is obviously a bad idea, but many parents do not realize that replacing the pop with "healthy" apple or orange juice is also loading the poor kids with fructose. High concentrations of fructose are found in fruit juice and in many soft drinks and sodas. These drinks are often sweetened with either sucrose (50 percent fructose) or high-fructose corn syrup (55 percent fructose). If rats are given fructose-rich drinks in addition to their normal food, they soon put on weight around the middle, a pattern similar to the metabolic syndrome associated in humans with diabetes, heart disease, and stroke.[18]

Both high-fructose corn syrup (HFCS) and sucrose are harmful and should be avoided. You need to read food labels in order to do this, as HFCS is found in many processed foods, including some you might not expect, such as bread, cereals, yogurt, and mayonnaise.

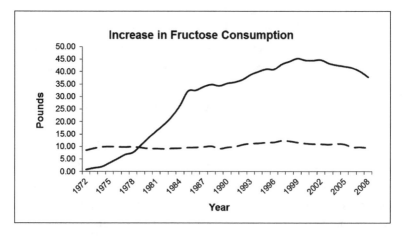

THE AVAILABILITY OF HIGH-FRUCTOSE CORN SYRUP (SOLID LINE) HAS INCREASED ALONG WITH THE RISE IN OBESITY SINCE ITS INTRODUCTION IN THE EARLY 1970S. THE INTAKE OF GLUCOSE (DASHED LINE) HAS REMAINED ABOUT CONSTANT. (DATA FROM USDA/ECONOMIC RESEARCH SERVICE, 2010.)

KEEPING YOU HUNGRY

Contrary to popular belief, consumption of carbohydrates is more dangerous than eating saturated fat or cholesterol. As we have seen, fructose or fruit sugar is particularly harmful. Common table sugar and HFCS contain similar amounts, although there is slightly more fructose in corn syrup and it is more rapidly absorbed. Furthermore, corn syrup can contain large amounts of additional breakdown toxins (called reactive carbonyls), particularly when stored in liquids at room temperature, such as in children's drinks. HFCS is even more fattening and damaging than sucrose. We need to be clear: fructose is poisonous. Sugar-laden sodas are not just empty calories—they are toxic.

Ancel Keys, who led the "cholesterol causes heart disease" campaign, misunderstood his results. The levels of saturated fat he measured were correlated with the subjects' intake of sugar, as well as with their levels of heart disease. A doughnut or a cookie, for example, consists of a combination of saturated fat and sugar. Such a combination is characteristic of processed and manufactured foods. When the population's intake of fat went up, so did their consumption of sugar. Keys simply ignored the sugar. If he had considered it, the world might not have been led on a wild goose (fat) chase.

Food containing saturated fat keeps you feeling full for longer than low-fat, sugar-rich meals. One reason low-carbohydrate diets work is that the presence of relatively high fat and protein levels leads to satiation. People eat less, because they are less hungry. Food manufacturers are aware that sugary foods are enticing, almost to the point of being addictive. Furthermore, since fructose will not increase your blood sugar, it does not inhibit the controls that should stop you eating in the same way that glucose does. Consider the popularity of colas sweetened with sugar or HFCS. Common forms of cola contain high levels of caffeine, sugar, and salt. These ingredients are diuretics: they increase your urine output, which makes you thirsty. The advantage to the cola companies is clear—the more cola you drink, the more you want to drink, and the more money they make!

A high-fructose diet will cause you to remain relatively hungry, while increasing your blood lipids and damaging your arteries. Eat some sugar and you will eat more. Over a time, it leads to deposition of belly fat and to metabolic syndrome. Fortunately, type 2 diabetes can be reversed by a simple change of diet. A Paleolithic diet that excludes grains, refined sugar, and processed oils will cure type 2 diabetes relatively quickly, perhaps within a month. This can be compared with the efforts of corporate medicine, which would place people with diabetes on a lifetime of drug maintenance.

IMPORTANT POINTS

- The focus on cholesterol and fats ignored the alternative explanation—that sugar was the culprit.

- Fructose or fruit sugar is implicated in heart disease, diabetes, and obesity.

- Table sugar (sucrose) and high-fructose corn syrup both contain fructose.

- Avoiding fructose can promote cardiovascular health.

- Glucose and many other sugars are relatively safe.

CHAPTER 6

RISK FACTORS AND INFLAMMATION

*"Science consists in grouping facts so that general
laws or conclusions may be drawn from them."*
—CHARLES DARWIN

Nowadays, nearly everyone knows the name of an obscure steroid called cholesterol. This is rather strange because few will have heard of substances such as carnosine or mevalonic acid. Although all three are essential to the normal functioning of the body, only one has become infamous. This happened because medicine became dominated by social science and statistics. Despite the claims for evidence-based medicine, epidemiology and clinical trials alone will not provide an explanation for cardiovascular disease or allow us to control it.

The medical profession's fascination with social studies and clinical trials restricts investigation into the direct cause of heart disease. Despite an enormous investment of scientific effort, research funding, and public education, progress has been slow. Researchers are describing increasing numbers of "risk factors," which tend to add further confusion, rather than helping to boost understanding.

If a cure for heart disease is to be found, we need to have a fundamental understanding of how and why heart attacks and strokes occur.[1] Basic science provides an explanation for cardiovascular disease in terms of inflammation and oxidation.

THE DEAD END OF SOCIAL SCIENCE

We have entered a new era of stagnation in medical research: social science and its associated statistics are supplanting basic investigation. Medical science has become a topsy-turvy world, where direct clinical observation is seen as secondary to large-scale statistical studies. Perhaps before assuming that experimental evidence is determined by statistics, medical researchers should remember the father of nuclear physics, Ernest Rutherford, the man who first split the atom. Rutherford warned, "If your result needs a statistician, then you should design a better experiment." His views on social science apply equally to epidemiology: "The only possible interpretation of any research whatever in the 'social sciences' is: some do, some don't."

What do we mean by "social science"? In this context, we mean the kind of research into heart disease that often involves large-scale population studies, to identify the relative importance of minor risk factors in the development of the illness. Clinical trials have also followed this approach—practical large-scale investigations with a disregard for direct clinical observation, individual variation, and theory. These types of studies, as opposed to basic experimental science, dominate medical research. Following on from this approach, prevention focuses on avoiding the resulting statistical risk factors.

To investigate heart disease, epidemiologists and other social scientists might examine the number and characteristics of people who have heart attacks. Certain factors, such as a particular environment, job hazards, family patterns, and specific personal habits are more prevalent in people who have suffered coronary thrombosis. People who are more prone to the disease, for example, might include overweight, middle-aged men who smoke and eat junk food. As a result of this research, we are bombarded with helpful—if sometimes conflicting—information about avoiding heart disease. The current model for good health is one in which people get regular exercise and eat a low-fat, low-salt diet that includes five daily helpings of fruits and vegetables. According to the health authorities, dietary supplementation is unnecessary if the person eats a normal, healthy diet.

Unfortunately, the majority of this well-meaning advice is based on weak evidence. People on these "healthy" diets who conform to these standard recommendations can still die prematurely of heart disease or stroke. As Rutherford might have put it, some die and some don't. Despite this, the authorities parade their recommendations as "proven" facts. Science, however, is not a collection of isolated facts—it is a systematic method for understanding the rules of nature. It could be that nonsmoking vegetarians who exercise are somewhat less likely to suffer premature death, but that is hardly comforting to the majority of people who, for whatever reason, are unable to stick to the recommendations.

The end result is a sequence of near-random pronouncements. There is no underlying theory: just a collection of *ex-cathedra* statements. Sometimes these disagree; for example, we have heard that "drinking coffee causes heart disease" and "drinking coffee can help prevent a heart attack." When conflicts occur, the defense is to talk about the reliability of the statistics or the size of the study.

Risk factors for cardiovascular disease are proclaimed in the press with regularity, but no rational explanation is offered. As we were writing this, it was announced that heart attacks are triggered by cold weather.[2] The study was considered reliable, as it met the requirements of evidence-based medicine, was performed by the London School of Hygiene and Tropical Medicine, and was published in the *British Medical Journal,* which is owned by the British Medical Association. Thus, this supposedly important study has an impressive stamp of approval from the authorities.

The study reported that a one-degree centigrade drop in temperature increases the risk of heart attack by 2 percent over the next month. This small increase was supposed to be important, because it might mean 200 new deaths in the United Kingdom, for example. However, the British population currently numbers about

59 million, which means that the risk to an individual person is insignificant. The increased chance of an individual Briton, chosen at random, having a heart attack following cold weather is about 1 in 300,000. A person worried about such a slight increase is at risk of being considered irrational.

Apparently, the BMJ report did not investigate whether wearing warm clothing or switching on the central heating would help to avoid this risk, although commentators suggested that this "obvious" intervention would be "unlikely to do you any harm."[3] Presumably, we need to wait until another large and expensive trial is performed to investigate whether keeping warm will modify the effects of cold weather or whether a woolen sweater might be superior to one made of acrylic. This sad situation typifies the use of so-called evidence-based medicine.

On average, people are eating more junk food, exercising less, and getting fatter. It is thus surprising that, since 1950, deaths from cardiovascular disease have been *falling*. The claimed risk factors do not explain the rise and fall of heart disease in the twentieth century.[4] Population studies do not tell us the cause of heart disease; for this, we need to understand its physiology and pathology. We need to consider what happens in an individual, rather than in a population.

FINDING CURES

Throughout the previous century, medical science made great strides in understanding the nature of diseases. Breakthroughs included insulin for diabetes, the beginnings of molecular biology, antibiotics, and advances in surgery. Since the 1950s, however, progress has slowed dramatically, with fewer groundbreaking treatments being discovered.

These days, advances in medical science tend to be imports from other disciplines. X-Ray computed tomography (CT) scans and magnetic resonance imaging (MRI) scans came from physics, for example. Sciences such as biochemistry and genetics have made steady progress, but this has not yet been translated into revolutionary new treatments. Dr. James Le Fanu, author of *The Rise and Fall of Modern Medicine,* has suggested that the introduction of social medicine, together with a gene-centric approach to disease, is responsible for this lack of progress. It is as if medical science has lost the knack of finding cures.

Epidemiology and large clinical trials can point the way, indicating that a relationship between cardiovascular disease and diet exists. On its own, however, social medicine does not provide a scientific explanation of that relationship. Similarly, epidemiology and statistics do not and cannot scientifically "prove" that a high-fat diet or other risk factor causes heart disease.

THE FRAMINGHAM STUDY

In 1948, the Framingham Heart Study was set up to identify the common factors that contribute to cardiovascular disease. Researchers recruited over 5,000 men and women between the ages of thirty and sixty-two from the town of Framingham, Massachusetts. The researchers tracked the subjects' health over a long period to see who might develop cardiovascular disease. The study was one of the biggest medical investigations of the twentieth century. Before Framingham, clinical investigations of heart disease were typically small or descriptive case reports.[5] In other words, they were the type of research that used to drive rapid medical progress.

In 1961, the initial report on risk factors in heart disease was published.[6] The results confirmed that high blood pressure, smoking, and high cholesterol levels were in some way associated with the disease. Framingham helped establish the risk factor concept and identified risks associated with heart disease and stroke, including obesity, diabetes, and physical inactivity. The researchers went on to recruit a second and then a third generation of participants. The study helped create a revolution in medicine: it changed the way medics and the general population viewed the origins of disease. Doctors considered the Framingham study a model for other longitudinal cohort studies. Furthermore, rather than looking for a predominant cause, doctors have been persuaded that heart disease is multi-factorial: in other words, it is caused by many factors, each contributing a little to the overall illness. This clearly makes treatment more complex than if the root cause is identified and addressed.

RISK FACTORS RATHER THAN CAUSES

The Framingham study generated risk factors for heart disease rather than causes. It could not show that such risk factors cause heart disease, as it was a study of the sociology of the illness, rather than its physiology or pathology. It may have demonstrated correlations, showing that links of some kind exist, but this is not sufficient to establish the cause. In 1947, Bradford Hill and Edward Kennaway of St. Bartholomew's Hospital, London, determined criteria that must be met before a causal link could be concluded. Rather than a vague statistical association, there needs to be additional direct evidence of a mechanism that causes the illness. The current risk factors do not meet these requirements.

There is no clear explanation for how risk factors cause atherosclerosis. Typically, the link between a risk factor and heart disease is relatively weak. In some studies, high cholesterol is associated with lower mortality and may be protective against atherosclerosis.[7] High blood cholesterol is weakly associated with heart attacks in young to middle-aged men. However, older people do not share this link between high cholesterol and mortality.[8] People with low blood cholesterol can have heart attacks,[9] and lowering cholesterol values may not save lives.[10] Low cholesterol may even be associated with higher death rates in some groups.[11] Finally, animal experiments have not shown that heart attacks occur due to increased cholesterol.[12] The cause lies elsewhere.

Imagine asking a mechanic why your clutch has failed and getting this reply: "It's multifactorial. We have noticed that Toyotas have more trouble than Fords, except for the 2008 Yaris, if

EVIDENCE BASED?

We are expected to believe that the new statistical medicine is "evidence-based" and provides a scientific way of keeping us healthy. The key to this approach is the determination of statistical risk factors. If we find the risk factors associated with heart disease, so the story goes, we can avoid them and remain healthy. It is assumed to be that simple.

The result might be amusing, if it were not causing so much harm. Hugh Davies compiled a list on Facebook of the "things that give you cancer."[13] These were risk factors that had been published by *The Daily Mail,* a leading newspaper in the United Kingdom. Typically, such articles draw on the latest medical research, although they are written in a popular manner. The A-to-Z of factors started with "age" and ran through "candlelit dinners," "gardens," and "water," concluding at x-rays. There were twenty-eight factors beginning with the letter *C*—definitely a letter to be avoided! Couples might be hard-pressed to avoid these risks since "sex," "children," and "childlessness" were all listed as causing cancer. Even reading the article itself was to be avoided, as using Facebook was on the list!

A second, derivative list was created on Facebook,[14] which was perhaps even funnier. Many of the entries had two links. The first link was to *The Daily Mail* article saying that a particular factor causes cancer, and the second to a report in the same paper, claiming it prevents cancer. So, for example, having a pet dog would both cause cancer ("a 29-fold increase"[15]) and lower the owner's risk of lymphoma by a third.[16] Technically, both these statements could be accurate, but to the typical reader they are simply confusing. Such reports are incomprehensible to the layperson and decision scientist alike.

So-called evidence-based medicine is bringing science into disrepute. Its methods are so questionable that it is held to ridicule, while corporate medicine regards it with a level of zeal normally reserved for fundamentalist religions.

yellow, red, or green with a go-faster stripe. Lack of a recent oil change and driving in the mountains are also correlated with the problem. Cars in the city are more at risk, and current evidence suggests an association with air pollution. Cars with tow bars also seem to have a high incidence; we suggest that tow bars are avoided and you use a rope when towing . . ." and so on. Most people would be astonished by such an answer: they would expect the mechanic to give a proper explanation. Surprisingly, people accept this kind of risk factor gibberish from a doctor, though they might consider others making similar statements to be irrational.

BACK TO BASICS

In order to understand what is going on in cardiovascular disease, we need to get back to basics. In the above example of a failed clutch, an automobile with a tow bar is more likely to wear out its clutch because it is subject to mechanical stress when the car is used to pull a heavy trailer. Ditching the tow bar for a rope, as our evidence-based mechanic suggested, is unlikely to prevent the stress on the clutch. Similarly, medicine needs to get back to cause and explanation, rather than mere statistical association, if it is to avoid equally fallacious cures.

Whenever medical problems such as heart disease are described in terms of risk factors, the biological understanding is deficient. However, finding new scientific explanations is exceedingly difficult: it relies on an individual scientist seeing through the tangle of risk factors and associations to provide a new model or theory. It is reassuring to remember that most medical problems eventually turn out to have a simple explanation.

We can sum up the evidence to date by saying that, although the conventional risk factors—such as smoking, high blood pressure, or a high-fat diet—may *contribute* to atherosclerosis in some way, they do not *cause* it. We know this because there are people who live a long life despite doing everything "wrong" in terms of the major risk factors. Conversely, a vegetarian who has a particular aversion to animal fats and cholesterol may still die from rampant atherosclerosis at a young age. The existence of such people, even if unusual, refutes the idea that the statistical factors cause heart disease or that avoiding these so-called risks will prevent it.

Risk factors apply to populations—they are rarely, if ever, accurate enough to predict the outcome in an individual. Even if we consider all the risk factors as a whole, they do not constitute the cause of heart disease. One objection to the suggestion that conventional risk factors fully explain heart disease is that genetic factors could also be involved. However, the changing incidence of heart disease in the last century is not explained or reflected in the traditional risk factors,[17] even when genetic factors are taken into account.

Modern medical research often focuses on genetics. Genes themselves are the basic units of heredity and consist of lengths of DNA (deoxyribonucleic acid). They provide the code for manufacturing enzymes and other proteins within the body's cells. Thus, genes and the way they express themselves—by assembling proteins—affect the body's biochemistry and physiology. Genetic changes occur over periods measured in generations, which makes them difficult to study. Furthermore, there are relatively few illnesses where a single gene demonstrably causes a particular disease. Illnesses caused by single faulty genes are rare. There is no gene for cancer or schizophrenia, for example. In most cases, many genes are thought to act as "risk factors"—somehow combining together to make the illness more likely.

Finding that a gene is associated with a disease may provide a pointer to an underlying biochemical problem. However, identifying the gene does not provide an automatic explanation or suggest a therapy. In the case of heart disease, suggesting the involvement of a genetic component simply means that some people are born with an abnormal biochemical constitution that may make them more susceptible. The important objective should be to determine the underlying physiological mechanisms and find out how these may be modified, to restore the person's health.

INFLAMMATION EXPLAINS THE RISK

Most risk factors for cardiovascular disease are linked with inflammation and oxidation. In other words, the risk factors can help initiate or prolong inflammation of the arteries. The list of factors linked with atherosclerosis is extensive and growing, and includes: disordered lipid profiles, such as high blood levels of LDL cholesterol; autoimmunity and infection; diabetes; and high blood levels of homocysteine.[18] Other risk factors include oxidative stress, genetic predisposition, asymmetrical dimethyl-arginine, C-reactive protein, and various metabolic diseases. It is interesting that most of these risk factors help fuel chronic inflammation.

The various risk factors can also act synergistically on different aspects of the inflammatory response mechanism, increasing their collective effects. They may stimulate the actions of immune cells, which respond to injury, and the release of molecules that are involved in inflammation. Inflammatory mediators include reactive oxygen species, such as nitric oxide, popularly recognized as oxidants. Often, they are simply things that we would expect to be associated with arterial stress, inflammation, or oxidation.

The conventional risk factors for atherosclerosis often affect three arterial cell types: endothelial cells, smooth muscle cells, and white blood cells.[19] Endothelial cells line the inner surface of the vessels, forming the boundary between the blood vessel and the blood, and controlling the flow of hormones and other chemicals through the vessel wall.[20] If the endothelial lining is damaged, the blood vessel wall can become compromised, so the body will attempt to repair it.

Deeper in the arterial wall, smooth muscle cells maintain the vessel's tone and structure. As we described earlier, the vascular tone describes the way the muscle cells in the wall contract and relax, decreasing or increasing blood flow, as required. If the smooth muscles cells are compromised (by sugars crosslinking proteins, for example), the vessel becomes less able to accommodate the pulsating blood flow from the heart. This can lead to high blood pressure and mechanical damage to the vessel.

The third affected group consists of white blood cells, which work together to defend our bodies against attack from bacteria, viruses, and other potential dangers. White blood cells can enter a blood vessel wall to help defend against chemical or biological threats. Damage to these cells by oxidized cholesterol can drive inflammation of the arterial wall.

Overall, the risk factors for heart disease are what might be expected in a person with inflamed arteries. For example, smoking and high blood pressure promote oxidation and inflammation in the arterial wall.[21] The table gives approximate values for the relative importance of some standard conventional risk factors for heart attacks in women.[22] These risk values are relative to a person's normal risk of heart disease, which would have a value of 1.

APPROXIMATE IMPORTANCE OF RISK FACTORS FOR HEART ATTACK		
RISK MARKER	RELATIVE RISK	RANGE
Lipoprotein(a)	1.2	0.6–1.8
Homocysteine	1.5	1.1–3.0
Total cholesterol	2.0	1.4–4.3
Low-density lipoprotein (LDL) cholesterol	2.1	1.3–4.5
Apolipoprotein B	3.3	1.5–6.2
Total cholesterol to high-density lipoprotein (HDL) ratio	3.4	1.7–5.0
C-reactive protein	3.9	2.1–7.2
C-reactive protein + total cholesterol to HDL ratio	5.7	3.7–7.2

These relative risks need careful explanation, as relative values can easily be confusing. Take the example of total cholesterol, which has a relative risk of 2. If a person has a 1 in 1,000 chance of having a heart attack this year, then a relative risk of 2 will double that risk, to 2 in 1,000. However, if their relative risk was 10, this would increase their risk from 1 in 1,000 to 10 in 1,000, which is the same as 1 in 100. For a dependable and important association, look for relative risks above 3 (preferably greater than 5). Larger evidence-based studies should have higher values, as they contain thousands of subjects and can show that an unimportant effect is statistically significant. Do not be fooled; treat all relative risk values with a pinch of salt.

Even if we assume that the values of these risks are accurate, their individual explanatory power is not great. Total cholesterol, for example, doubles a small risk. The largest single factor is C-reactive protein, with a relative risk of almost 4. C-reactive protein is a specific indicator of inflammation.

RESEARCH HYPE

With medicine as social science, clinical trials are used to show that in a group of people taking a drug, such as a statin, the drug lowers an average risk factor, such as cholesterol levels. These results are then used to give advice and treatment, or to attempt to prevent disease.

At the heart of this approach lies a well-established problem, which researchers ignore. Clinical trials aim to tell whether the response of one group of people differs in some way from that of a second group. A clinical trial might show that, on average, a drug will prevent heart attacks. However, this result does not apply to a particular individual. Giving people an average medical treatment in this way is as irrational as asking a whole population to wear shoes of an average size: most people would be very uncomfortable, as their new shoes would be either too big or too small—individuals are not average, they are different.

A statin drug might be found to slightly lower the average risk of heart attack, but the number of patients who need to be treated to prevent a single heart attack may be in the region of 100. Thus, ninety-nine of the people taking the drug will not benefit, but they will be required to pay for the treatment and to risk its side effects.

STATINS AND THEIR HIDDEN SIDE EFFECTS

First a warning: if you decide to use statins, you may not retain enough brain power to come off them! This may be an overstatement but, although clinical trials frequently claim low levels of side effects, patients on these cholesterol-lowering drugs have reported memory loss, clouded thinking, and confusion. Gradually, these warnings are entering the mainstream media.[23]

Duane Graveline, a medical doctor and former NASA astronaut, has written several books about his disturbing experiences with statin drugs.[24] After he was prescribed statins, Dr. Graveline experienced transient global amnesia; this meant that, for a short time, he lost his memory. As he explains, "For twelve hours, I was a thirteen-year-old high school student who knew my subjects, teachers, and every kid in my class (according to my worried wife), but with no memory for my entire adult life." Graveline stopped taking the statins and investigated their side effects. He soon realized he had been pretty lucky. Other statin victims had reported suffering neuromuscular problems, short-term memory loss, Parkinson-like symptoms, and amyotrophic lateral sclerosis (ALS)—a progressive and fatal neurological disease.

The side effects popularly reported for statins are at odds with reports from clinical trials. This is not particularly surprising, as clinical trials are of short duration and a side effect may take some time to show itself. During clinical trials, researchers look out for side effects to estimate the safety of a drug. Despite this, even obvious problems, such as thalidomide limb shortening, can go unreported until a drug has been on the market for years. In addition, the patient may not realize that his or her symptoms have anything to do with the drug; many people expect to be more forgetful as they age, for example. Some patients on statins fear they are becoming demented or might have Alzheimer's disease, because their memory is fading. Other reported side effects, such as muscle weakness, might also be attributed to increasing age.

Guidelines for patient safety indicate that statins may cause sleep disruption, memory loss, sexual disturbances, inflammation of the lungs, and depression.[25] These side effects would only be worth suffering if the benefits were large and substantial. Although the standard claim is that statin drugs prevent more than 30 percent of heart attacks, this is misleading.

The table below shows how many people must be treated to help a single patient; this is the "number needed to treat" (NNT). The figures imply that 107 people should take statins for a year to prevent one death. In other words, 107 patients would need to be treated, at a combined cost of around $100,000, to have a reasonable chance of saving one life. The chance of the drug saving a particular person's life is correspondingly remote (about 1 in 100). These figures have been taken from *Bandolier,* an independent journal about evidence-based health care,[26] and may be regarded as optimistic.

NUMBER OF PEOPLE WHO MUST TAKE STATINS TO PREVENT ONE DEATH OR ILLNESS	
EVENT	NUMBER NEEDED TO TREAT (NNT)
Death from all causes	107
All strokes	330
All coronary heart disease (CHD)	48
All strokes plus all CHD	42

Based on these and similar data, statins hardly appear the wonder drugs they are claimed to be. The next table gives the figures for patients who have already suffered cardiovascular events. These are slightly more encouraging, though better results can be achieved with good nutrition and supplements. Moreover, patients want a drug with a number needed to treat (NNT) close to 1. They want a good chance that they will gain from the drug, not to waste money making up the numbers, for someone else to benefit.

NUMBER OF PEOPLE WITH CARDIOVASCULAR DISEASE WHO MUST TAKE STATINS TO PREVENT ONE DEATH OR ILLNESS	
EVENT	NUMBER NEEDED TO TREAT (NNT)
All cause death	33
All strokes	71
All heart attacks (coronaries)	14
All strokes and coronaries	12

As the side effects of statins become more apparent, the measured risk of harm is likely to increase. Some already put the risk of harm at one in five patients. Dr. Malcolm Kendrick, author of *The Cholesterol Con,* disputes that the benefits outweigh the advantages: "Even if a man who had a heart attack, and was at high risk of another, took statins for forty years, he would only extend his life by just 17.5 days. Is it really worth putting up with all those side effects for that?"[27] Those 17.5 days would cost the man something in the region of $40,000, which could have been used more effectively on preventive nutrition, perhaps using the remainder for an ocean cruise and other long vacations.

The kind of mistake that wrongly attributes conclusions from research on groups to individuals is called the ecological fallacy. We can paraphrase it by saying that the results of a large-scale clinical trial or epidemiological study are often of little or no importance to the treatment of an individual patient. A risk factor for a population does not necessarily apply directly to you!

Gradually, the public is becoming aware that there is a problem with modern medical research. Clinical trials face increasing public distrust, as claims are often contradictory.[28] For years, people were advised to take an aspirin a day to prevent heart attacks. Then, a clinical trial showed that aspirin is bad for you, as it can cause internal bleeding and increase your risk of stroke. Similarly, we were told to avoid the midday sun—it might cause skin cancer or make us look old before our time. But more recently, doctors have begun to advise us to spend more time in the sun to increase levels of vitamin D and thereby prevent cancer. The option to take a vitamin D supplement is mostly ignored. As this book was being written, a report suggested that the healthiest start to the day was a fried breakfast of bacon, sausages, eggs, and beans.[29] After years of advice on avoiding cholesterol and fat, who can blame anyone for feeling confused?

In science, the important experiments have a simplicity and elegance. The result is a definite observation or measurement, which is easy to reproduce. Since corporate medicine adopted social science and statistics as an alternative, the results are diffuse, contradictory, and unconvincing. The studies are also too large and expensive to be easily replicated. People in the United States are becoming particularly distrustful of pharmaceutical companies and most believe that drug companies put profits ahead of patients' interests.[30]

The medical profession considers clinical trials as their gold standard and accepts them as "proof" of a treatment's efficacy. A treatment is referred to as "clinically proven" or even "scientifically proven" when it has passed the test of at least one large-scale, randomized trial. Unfortunately, most of these trials report biased or incorrect information. The quasi-legal jargon is misleading, because if a doctor thinks a medical idea is "proven," there is no need to look beyond it. Thus, further research or investigation is stifled.

Equally important, treatments that have not been subject to randomized, placebo-controlled clinical trials of sufficient size may be denigrated as "unproven." While this unscientific slur may be technically correct, it applies to all science, which is inductive. There is no such thing as scientific proof! Unproven does not mean the treatment does not work. A more apt description would be "untested," since proof is a legal concept rather than a scientific one. Just because an idea has not attracted the resources to carry out large-scale trials does not mean it is wrong. It may be a wonderful, long-sought cure, but one that cannot offer enough potential profits to make testing it financially worthwhile.

A valuable and inexpensive solution to heart disease may have already been found and ignored. Unless governments (who should stand to benefit from cost-effective improvements to health) take responsibility for testing such treatments, we will not have the chance to find out.

IMPORTANT POINTS

- The aim of science is to explain how the world works – cause and effect.

- The promotion of risk factors for heart disease indicates ignorance of the cause.

- "Proven" and "unproven" are legal terms rather than scientific concepts.

- Risk factors do not indicate an individual's chance of having a heart attack or stroke.

- The current risk factors suggest inflammation of the arteries.

- The solution to the epidemic of cardiovascular disease is to prevent or treat arterial inflammation.

CHAPTER 7

OVERLOOKED EVIDENCE

"Men, it has been well said, think in herds;
it will be seen that they go mad in herds,
while they only recover their senses slowly,
and one by one."
—CHARLES MACKAY (1814–1889),
EXTRAORDINARY POPULAR DELUSIONS
AND THE MADNESS OF CROWDS

Perhaps the surprising thing about the description of atherosclerosis as inflammation is how long it has taken to become the dominant scientific model. Inflammation was identified as the major issue over a century ago, though corporate medicine seems to have disregarded its relevance to heart disease. Inflammation is the body's response to damage and infection. Any chemical, mechanical, or immunological damage to an artery triggers a cascade of inflammatory processes aimed at local repair.[1] Almost all of the traditional risk factors for heart disease can play minor roles in triggering or supporting local areas of inflammation.

The connection between heart disease and inflammation suggests approaches to treatment and prevention, particularly the use of anti-inflammatories and antioxidants. Substances that aid tissue repair may also be useful. The following section describes examples of potentially effective solutions to cardiovascular disease, some of which may have been overlooked for several decades.

THE PIONEERING WORK OF
LESTER MORRISON

Health journalist Bill Sardi recently reminded people of the work of Dr. Lester Morrison, a pioneer in heart disease research.[2] Morrison's thought-provoking book suggested a potential cure for atherosclerosis and heart attacks.[3] The book's title, *Coronary Heart Disease and the Mucopolysaccharides (Glycosaminoglycans)*, was unlikely to make it a bestseller. While the obscure title may explain why few members of the public are aware of the book, it might be expected that the medical profession would have investigated the proposed treatment. Despite this, the book is largely forgotten and the medical establishment has ignored Morrison's research.

In the 1940s, Morrison was studying diet and heart disease. His own family suffered badly: his parents and several other relatives succumbed to the disease. In 1950, Morrison and his assistant, Kenneth Johnson, measured the cholesterol deposited in the arterial walls of people who had died from coronary artery disease. He found that, on average, they had four times as much cholesterol in their arteries as did controls, and they also tended to have higher blood levels.[4] At first Morrison concluded that the body's fat control mechanisms had changed in people with heart disease. Death from heart attack was thought to be a long process, starting at birth and progressing through childhood to ultimately threaten the middle-aged. By 1955, however, he realized that atherosclerosis involved more than the arteries wearing out as a result of age and stress.[5] In those early years, it had not been realized that the accumulated damage was a result of a failure to repair the initial injuries. Like modern researchers, Morrison was able to identify factors that were associated with coronary disease, including diet, certain drugs, sex hormones, blood coagulation, smoking, and local stress in the arterial walls. While there has been some detailed clarification, little has fundamentally changed in the identification of major risk factors since that time.

Dr. Morrison was interested in dietary modifications that might prevent heart disease. In 1949, he reported an experiment with choline,[6] which is found in lecithin, a food supplement. He studied 115 patients who had suffered a heart attack. Patients were given 12 grams of choline a day. This large dose was taken for one year by fifty-two patients, for two years by thirty-five patients, and for three years by twenty-eight patients. Thus, the supplement was given for between one and three years, after recovery from heart attack. He compared the results with another 115 control patients, who had suffered heart attacks but were not given choline. The choline appeared to save lives: thirty-five control patients died, whereas only fourteen of the supplemented patients died.

In 1960, based on the idea that cholesterol causes heart disease, Morrison modified the diets of patients with coronary atherosclerosis: fifty patients were put on a low-fat, low-cholesterol diet; the other fifty patients were controls, who were not given the treatment. Twelve years later, nineteen of the patients on the low-fat diet had survived, but all controls had passed away.[7] This is a convincing demonstration that changing the diet can prolong survival in patients with coronary disease. The obvious implication is that lowering dietary fat can reduce the number of deaths in people suffering from coronary disease. However, this conclusion is too hasty; it was not necessarily the limitation of fat and cholesterol that caused the improvement—it could have been something that was substituted for them. Lowering the fat intake modified the whole diet. The total fat intake in the modified diet was 25 grams a day, and few animal fats were eaten. This implies that the change involved a fundamentally different diet and a variety of nutrients. Morrison suggested that a large statistical trial might evaluate the role of fat in coronary heart disease. Multiple such trials have been performed over the following decades, but have failed to show the same dramatic results. Fat is not the problem.

Shortly after his demonstration that changing the diet could save lives, Morrison published a remarkable paper,[8] which showed that he retained a willingness to consider alternative ideas—a trait all too rare in later medical researchers. In the 1950s, published reports suggested that chondroitin, a well-known food supplement used in the treatment of arthritis, could prevent atherosclerosis. Morrison's research team spent a year in the early 1960s studying sixty-five squirrel monkeys (*Saimiri sciurea*). These monkeys suffered a form of spontaneous atherosclerosis, which the researchers attempted to aggravate by feeding them an abnormal diet containing large amounts of cholesterol and butter. The monkeys were separated into six groups for investigation, three of which were given injections of chondroitin sulfate.

Chondroitin was found to lower the blood lipid levels in monkeys that had been given the cholesterol and butter diet. Of particular importance was Morrison's finding that cholesterol levels were also lower inside the aorta, the main artery leaving the heart. This implied that the animals' arteries were less diseased. Close visual examination of the aortas also suggested that animals treated with chondroitin had healthier arteries. Morrison realized that chondroitin sulfate might moderate or even prevent atherosclerosis.

By 1971, Morrison was aware of the evidence that chondroitin sulfate and related substances helped protect and heal the arteries. His choice of supplement was not random: chondroitin is an essential component of connective tissue, which helps "glue" the body tissues together. Connective tissues are found in tendons, ligaments, and joints. Tendons act like ropes, connecting muscles to bones, and their fibers are made of a protein called collagen, embedded in a gel-like material. This gel-like ground substance in connective tissue contains chondroitin, glucosamine, and hyaluronic acid, which are all known as supplements for arthritis. Dr. Morrison described these supplements as "the glue of life."

Reasoning that chondroitin, glucosamine, and hyaluronic acid might strengthen arteries and help them to heal, Morrison suggested that these substances could help prevent the arterial degeneration found in coronary disease.[9] In addition, they can also aid in preventing blood clotting, which ultimately causes heart attacks. By 1973, he had become convinced of the efficacy of chondroitin sulfate for preventing atherosclerosis and heart attack.[10] In 1975,

Morrison was granted a United States patent on the use of chondroitin sulfate in treatment of heart disease.[11] He suggested 500 to 10,000 milligrams of chondroitin sulfate should be taken daily in divided doses, with meals.

Morrison also described experiments on rats that, like the squirrel monkeys, were fed an abnormal diet that caused a form of atherosclerosis. Eighteen control rats were fed this diet, and sixteen of them survived but were found to have developed atherosclerotic plaques in their aortas. In the treatment group, eighteen rats received the same abnormal diet but with additional chondroitin. Only three of the eighteen were affected by aortic plaques. Similarly, the untreated rats all showed atherosclerosis of the coronary arteries, while only five of the chondroitin-treated group developed such lesions.

Similar results were reported with human heart patients. Of sixty control patients, twenty-nine had "events"; of these, sixteen were heart attacks, ten of which were fatal. Eight patients developed acute coronary insufficiency (inadequate blood flow to the heart) and five suffered milder ischemia. Out of sixty patients treated with chondroitin, only four had events, though all were fatal. Of these, three suffered fatal heart attacks and one developed coronary insufficiency. Chondroitin appeared to save lives. Furthermore, Morrison found that of the treated patients who had suffered heart attacks, two had not taken their chondroitin according to schedule: one stopped taking it two months before dying; the second took it only intermittently for a year. The patient with

TRIAL OF CHONDROITIN IN CARDIAC PATIENTS					
GROUP	HEART ATTACK		INSUFFICIENCY	ISCHEMIA	TOTAL
	FATAL	NON-FATAL			
Controls	4 men, 2 women	6 men, 4 women	4 men, 4 women	0 Men, 5 women	14 men, 15 women
Treated	2 men, 1 woman	0 men, 0 women	0 men, 1 woman	0 men, 0 women	2 men, 2 women

insufficiency also had uncontrollably high blood pressure and died of a stroke. At autopsy, only one of the deaths could be reliably attributed to failure of the treatment.

These results were reported by Morrison over a period of three years. Three years later, eight more deaths had occurred in the control group, but none in the treated group. Thus, there were 14 deaths in the controls and only 3 in those receiving chondroitin. Between 1942 and 1955, Dr. Morrison's results with 134 patients treated with chondroitin were remarkable:

- Coronary arteriosclerotic heart disease—74 percent improved

- Arteriosclerosis of the brain arteries—77 percent improved

- Arteriosclerosis in the legs—80 percent improved

Morrison became convinced of the benefits of chondroitin: "The results were more than good, they were marvelous." He described chondroitin as the "coronary artery's first line of defense against invasion by foreign substances." These results suggest that supplements of chondroitin sulfate might protect millions of people from atherosclerosis and heart attack. If these results are correct, a simple, low-cost chondroitin supplement could save the lives of many those individuals who already have the disease.

Astonishingly, despite Morrison's dramatic research results, high-dose chondroitin was not subjected to repeated clinical trials to either confirm or deny that it could largely eradicate coronary thrombosis. Instead, the results were ignored. Indeed, by 1990, chondroitin sulfate was being implicated in the pathology of atherosclerosis.[12] Some people thought the presence of chondroitin in arterial plaques was harmful rather than helpful, as it attracts cholesterol. Once again, a fixation on the idea that cholesterol is the culprit in heart disease may have diverted attention from a potential cure.

Morrison's results make physiological sense. When damaged, an artery responds by repairing the tissue and strengthening its wall. Since atherosclerosis is inflammation of the artery wall, the process of healing might well result in increased deposition of collagen, chondroitin sulfate, and other connective tissue components. This means that, far from being a cause of atherosclerosis, chondroitin may be used to repair the wall of the damaged vessel. An injured artery will respond by laying down connective tissue, including chondroitin, to strengthen itself. In this way, chondroitin and related substances accumulate in atherosclerotic plaque.[13] As might be expected, collagen levels are also increased.[14] Notably, chondroitin is an anti-inflammatory agent and helps inhibit local inflammation.[15]

AN ALTERNATIVE APPROACH

In looking for a cure to heart disease and stroke, we need to return to basics. Atherosclerosis starts with a minor disruption of the blood vessel wall. As explained earlier, such damage may be inflicted by the normal wear-and-tear of arterial flexing, associated with increased blood pressure, or even by the shear stress of blood as it pulses through the vessel, like a river eroding its banks.

If we are correct and atherosclerosis follows from mechanical damage, then the much larger trauma associated with cardiovascular surgery should lead to a massive increase in local atherosclerosis and, indeed, this is what happens. Organ transplant surgery is associated with increased atherosclerosis and may act as a model for the natural occurrence of the disease.[18] This model incorporates mechanical damage to the tissues, together with increased liability to infection, oxidation, and inflammation.

The inside of arteries is lined by endothelial cells, which separate the blood from the arterial wall. This lining is the first part of the artery to be damaged in atherosclerosis. The endothelial cells sense the current conditions and generate signals that control the response of the artery.[19] Damage to these cells plays a central part in triggering atherosclerosis.[20] The involvement of endothelial cells at the start of the disease means they are vital to our

IS MY CHOLESTEROL TOO HIGH?

The short answer is probably not. There is little evidence supporting the idea that high cholesterol will cause a person to have a
heart attack. Despite this, the idea that high cholesterol is harmful and causes atherosclerosis has resulted in an industry of testing and cholesterol-lowering foods and drugs. An important but
overlooked fact is that low cholesterol levels can be harmful.

Some of the official advice is absurd. There is little connection
between dietary intake and blood levels: the human body manufactures cholesterol in the liver and regulates its own blood
levels. Despite this, the American Heart Association (AHA) recommends that people control their intake of cholesterol.[16] According to the AHA, a person should eat less than 300 milligrams of
cholesterol a day; there is more than that in a large chicken egg!

The AHA's low-density lipoprotein (LDL) blood level recommendations are as follows:

- Optimal: 100 mg/dl

- Near or above optimal: 100–129 mg/dl

- Borderline high: 130–159 mg/dl

- High: 160–189 mg/dl

- Very high: 190 mg/dl

   For total cholesterol, the AHA's recommendations are:

- Desirable: Less than 200 mg/dl

- Borderline: high risk: 200–239 mg/dl

- High risk: More than 240 mg/dl

   In reality, unless your total cholesterol level is greater than
about 300 mg/dl, the "risk" is probably low. As we have stressed,
cholesterol levels do not *cause* heart attacks—they are simply
associated with them. People with low cholesterol can suffer

heart attacks, in addition to a range of related illnesses. Conversely, a person with massively high cholesterol may never develop atherosclerosis, heart disease, or stroke. Lowering your cholesterol may not lower your true risk of heart disease.

There is insufficient data to support the AHA's recommendations.[17] The authors of this book have never had a cholesterol test, have no intention of having one, and would be more concerned to find their total cholesterol level was below 100 mg/dl than above 300 mg/dl. Medicine has failed to cure heart disease and has turned cholesterol into an illness, as a smoke screen to cover this failure. To the contrary, however, there is little doubt that cholesterol is essential to good health.

understanding of heart disease and, ultimately, to discovering ways to control this illness. When damage occurs, the cells lining the artery send signals to start an inflammatory response.[21] They also release factors that affect blood clotting.[22] Endothelial cells govern the flow of nutrients to the artery wall and are intimately involved in the initiation of inflammation. They are biochemically active and release local hormones, such as nitric oxide, that signal the smooth muscle cells to maintain blood vessel tone and blood flow.[23]

The Role of Nitric Oxide

Nitric oxide (NO) is a simple molecule that maintains healthy blood vessels and prevents atherosclerosis.[24] It plays a central role in normal physiology and in disease processes, including inflammation, infection, and regulation of blood pressure.[25] Glyceryl trinitrite (GTN), which is a diluted form of the explosive nitroglycerin, acts by stimulating the release of nitric oxide to prevent angina. Nitric oxide expands blood vessels and promotes blood flow. The drug Viagra (sildenafil citrate) releases nitric oxide and was first studied as an anti-angina drug. Its action on erectile disfunction was an unexpected side effect. A related novel use for glyceryl trinitrite is its addition to the end of a condom—to stimulate erection, rather than an explosive event!

When concentrated, nitroglycerin is a highly unstable explosive; it will detonate if knocked, making it difficult to transport. Once the reaction has started, the compression wave travels at supersonic speed, detonating any further unstable material it encounters. Such high explosives show the energetic nature of redox reactions: an explosion is a heat-generating oxidation reaction that propagates so fast that it grows exponentially. This reactivity illustrates the power of oxidation and the need to curb it. While redox reactions are essential to the normal functioning of biological systems, they need extensive control systems for their regulation. Thankfully, our cells are not exposed to explosive oxidation but rather to the slow burning of aging and inflammation.

Damage to the body's synthesis of nitric oxide may be one of the first steps leading to atherosclerosis.[26] NO is formed from the amino acid arginine[27] and also involves vitamins B_2 (riboflavin) and B_3 (niacin).[28] Under the oxidizing conditions in inflamed tissues, superoxide can be produced instead of NO.[29] The potentially harmful superoxide generated by white blood cells can prevent NO from stimulating the local arterial wall to relax and dilate. As inflammation develops, superoxide will constrict local blood vessels, further antagonizing the action of nitric oxide.

Once formed, nitric oxide can spread rapidly through the endothelial cell membrane into the smooth muscle, helping to relax the arterial wall.[30] It provides a chemical signal, controlling both local blood flow and blood pressure[31]. It dilates the vessel and increases blood flow, so it is often considered antagonistic to hormones such as adrenaline.[32] Release of NO from endothelial cells can lessen injury from reduced blood flow by expanding the blood vessel. The increased blood flow can compensate for mild atherosclerosis. In advanced atherosclerosis, arteries may produce less nitric oxide, which may be related to the presence of local oxidation and free radicals.[33] Low levels of NO in tissues or decreased sensitivity to its effects can impair the ability of arteries to dilate when needed. The result is that atherosclerosis is more likely to result in clinical illness.[34] Nitric oxide helps prevent symptoms of cardiovascular disease.

In 1998, the importance of nitric oxide was acknowledged when the Nobel Prize in Medicine was awarded to Dr. Louis Ignarro for his work on NO's role in the cardiovascular system. It is not surprising, then, that NO is accepted as one of the more important local hormones regulating vascular tone and blood flow. In 2003, Ignarro suggested that atherosclerotic plaques act like trash caught in a river bend, impeding the flow. The result is local stress on the epithelial wall of the artery. When a blood vessel wall is stressed or damaged, its epithelial cells increase production of nitric oxide.[35] The generation of NO is initiated by several disparate chemical and mechanical factors, such as the sheer stress of the blood flowing against the arterial wall.[36] The realization that nitric oxide has these important properties suggests a possible solution to heart disease.

ARGININE AND ANTIOXIDANTS TO PREVENT ATHEROSCLEROSIS

Ignarro proposed a new approach to preventing atherosclerosis, heart disease, and stroke. His experiments suggested that dietary supplements of antioxidant vitamins and L-arginine, an amino acid found in the normal diet, could lower the risk of heart disease in mice.[37] People who have defective nitric oxide responses suffer thickening of the blood vessel wall and increased resistance to blood flow.[38] In order to model atherosclerosis, Ignarro used mice with a genetic defect in cholesterol metabolism, although he expected that his experiments would produce similar results in people with heart disease.[39] Based on his research, Ignarro suggested that arginine supplements would prevent atherosclerosis. However, this suggestion remains controversial.

Nitric oxide's involvement in maintaining the health of arteries suggests several nutritional approaches to the prevention of cardiovascular disease. In people with high blood pressure, high cholesterol, or high homocysteine levels, arginine supplementation can improve the ability of the arteries to expand. Conversely, blocking the action of nitric oxide contributes to free-radical damage, diabetes, and high cholesterol.[40]

Briefly, the role of arginine in protecting the blood vessels from damage suggests another physiological link between most conventional risk factors.[41] The obstruction of nitric oxide production in the blood vessels could explain many of the classic atherosclerosis risk factors, including high cholesterol, high blood pressure,[42] homocysteinemia,[43] kidney failure, heart failure,[44] and Reynaud's disease.[45] Conventional risk factors for heart disease, including high blood lipids, diabetes, high blood pressure, and smoking,[46] aging, diabetes, and insulin resistance are also linked, and can impair the ability of blood vessels to expand.[47] This explanation provides some degree of synthesis among the otherwise unrelated statistical factors.

Using arginine supplements alongside folic acid[48] and other B vitamins may be particularly beneficial. Antioxidants, such as vitamins C, E, and alpha-lipoic acid can also reduce oxidative stress and facilitate the action of NO.[49]

Arginine for Angina and Heart Failure

Given the role of nitric oxide in smooth muscle relaxation, arginine supplementation might help alleviate the symptoms of angina. Angina is chest pain resulting from stiffened or partly blocked arteries, which cannot supply enough blood to the heart muscle. In a study of ten people with intractable angina that was unresponsive to standard treatments, seven subjects showed improvement with daily supplements (9 grams) of arginine over a period of three months.[50] However, subjects with stable angina did not show improvement with arginine at higher (15 gram) doses.[51] A further trial of twenty-two subjects with stable angina following a heart attack indicated that 6 grams of arginine daily increased their exercise capacity.[52] A second study at this dose confirmed improvement in exercise tolerance.[53] The beneficial effects may relate to arterial expansion from increased nitric oxide.[54] Considering that in angina the vessels supplying the heart are typically atherosclerotic and diseased, a variable clinical response might be anticipated.

Arginine has been considered as a potential treatment for congestive heart failure, in which the heart becomes less effective at maintaining blood flow through the tissues. Once again, increasing nitric oxide in the tissues could cause blood vessels to dilate, increasing blood flow. Trials of arginine supplementation in patients with heart failure showed increased blood flow compared with a placebo,[55] as well as improved kidney function.[56] Even though research is at an early stage, looking at arginine is a far more productive approach than the research into the "risks" of too much cholesterol.

Clinical Trials?

There is currently limited clinical information on the effects of arginine by itself in heart attack patients. One trial of arginine in patients who had suffered a heart attack was stopped because of an apparently increased death rate in the treated group.[57] However, stopping a trial makes it difficult to analyse the results. In this case, patients in the treatment group supplemented with 3 grams of arginine, three times a day. Of 177 patients in the trial, five in the treatment group died within six months, compared with none in the placebo group. However, in two of the five patients, death was caused by sepsis rather than heart disease and a further two were found dead at home and the cause of death was not determined. The recommendation was that arginine should not be used following a heart attack; this conclusion was premature.

Prof. Rainer Böger of the University of Hamburg, Germany,

criticized this study, noting that arginine has a short half-life in the blood plasma.[58] Half of the arginine absorbed would be lost from the blood within an hour. However, there is a more serious objection to the study. Arginine was found to have increased more in the blood of the control patients than the treated patients who received large doses! We suggest that the researchers might have reevaluated their experimental methods to understand this anomaly. One issue with supplement trials is that sick people in the control group may elect to self-supplement, if they know what is happening. Moreover, since the blood levels overlapped, we do not understand how the researchers could reach the conclusion that the arginine was responsible for anything at all.

A larger study indicated fewer deaths with arginine supplementation.[59] In 792 patients, heart attack (myocardial ischemia) occurred in 24 percent of the treated patients and 27 percent of those receiving placebo. The arginine had no serious side effects. Thus, the two studies mentioned were contradictory. A later review of both studies concluded that arginine had no effect on heart attack patients.[60] However, we consider there were insufficient data to reach a conclusion on the benefits or otherwise.

We find these trials inconclusive and a little misleading. Giving such a large dose of arginine by itself is inappropriate as a supplement strategy. In a clinical trial, a large dose of a single supplement has merit, as it helps to find out the effects of the substance. However, this does not have great relevance to a person wanting to use supplements to avoid a heart attack or stroke. A more sensible approach is perhaps 1 gram or so of arginine taken between meals, along with a large dose of antioxidants, particularly vitamin C. This is closer to Ignarro's recommendation.

Antioxidant Defenses in Plaque

The main cause of the chronic inflammation in atherosclerosis is a shortage of antioxidants. In 1955, Dr. G.C. Willis discovered that vitamin C depletion is common in human arteries, where high

SAY "YES" TO NO!

Atherosclerosis has been described as an arginine deficiency disease. Arginine is a semi-essential amino acid (it is not considered an essential amino acid, as it can be synthesized in the body).[61] However, body levels largely reflect the amount in the diet.[62] Deficiency of arginine from an inadequate diet could be common.

Arginine with vitamin C was promoted as a potential cure for atherosclerosis by Louis Ignarro, who won the 1998 Nobel Prize in Medicine. He recommended eating a diet high in antioxidants, arginine, and two other amino acids, citruline and taurine. Dr. Ignarro's 2006 book *NO More Heart Disease: How Nitric Oxide Can Prevent—Even Reverse—Heart Disease and Strokes* details how the work on nitric oxide (NO) that won him the Nobel Prize led him to believe that atherosclerosis could be prevented or even cured with nutritional supplements. He suggested that nitric oxide could expand blood vessels, lower cholesterol, and control platelets and blood clotting. If correct, NO would prevent heart attacks and many strokes. Additionally, he claims that increasing nitric oxide would reduce arterial plaques by 50 percent. This action depends on NO acting as an antioxidant.

The two main antioxidants in Ignarro's approach are vitamin C and alpha-lipoic acid. (Incidentally, Ignarro is the third Nobel Prize winner to suggest that high doses of vitamin C could protect against heart disease.) These nutrients are combined with arginine which, in addition to its role as the precursor for NO,[63] has a range of direct effects on the body, including stimulation of hormone release.[64] This may in part explain its action as a modulator of immune function and inflammation. This role has led to the investigation of arginine at doses of several grams per day in cancer therapy.[65]

If arginine is so important in maintaining the health of blood vessels, supplementing with this amino acid might be beneficial, particularly if it is taken with an antioxidant. Arginine has been shown to inhibit plaque formation and arterial thickening in some animal studies.[66] In patients with a deficiency of nitric oxide production, vitamin E may improve vascular function.[67] However, in clinical trials, the effectiveness of arginine has been inconsistent.[68] It may be that the main effect of arginine is preventive, because of NO's role in the early stages of arterial damage. A substance that prevents an illness may not necessarily make a clinically effective treatment, once the disease has become established.

Arginine is a normal component of the diet and is considered nontoxic. Typical doses of arginine are in the range of 1–3 grams per day, preferably taken with an equal or greater amount of vitamin C. However, people with a current herpes infection should refrain from high-dose supplementation, as the amino acid may aggravate their condition.[69]

levels would protect against oxidation.[70] Human plaque might actually contain more antioxidants than are found in healthy arteries; however, these antioxidants are quickly used up. In plaques, both vitamin E and coenzyme Q_{10} (CoQ_{10}) become oxidized.[71] The inflamed tissue may attempt to take up other antioxidants, but the quantity is not enough to prevent damage.

Vitamin E and CoQ_{10} are antioxidants that require a constant re-supply of electrons in order to prevent free radical damage. These antioxidants work by giving up electrons to stop free radical reactions and oxidation. Under the inflammatory conditions within a plaque, the abnormal metabolism is insufficient to provide enough antioxidant electrons. If nitric oxide is to protect the blood vessels, a high level of antioxidants may be essential. When tissue levels of oxidants are high, as in inflamed arterial wall, NO production may be high, but ineffective. Local oxidants inactivate the molecule before it can perform its physiological functions, such as increasing blood flow.[72] Also, while we have emphasized the need for sufficient NO, very high levels can be pathological, killing cells and generating free radical damage.[73] The benefits of nitric oxide depend on having sufficient antioxidants.

Several antioxidants have the potential to quench free radicals and preserve nitric oxide's beneficial function. These include vitamin E,[74] alpha-lipoic acid,[75] CoQ_{10},[76] glutathione,[77] superoxide dismutase (SOD),[78] selenium,[79] and quercetin.[80] Unfortunately, contrary to the popular misconception, these dietary antioxidants are typically not powerful enough to prevent or reverse atherosclerosis. Although they enter the inflamed plaque and help support NO, they are quickly used up. When this happens, they cease to be effective as antioxidants and play little role in stopping progression of the disease. If this were not so, then simply taking antioxidant supplements, some CoQ_{10} for example, would stop people having a heart attack. It would be easy to eliminate the disease. Typical antioxidants such as CoQ_{10} and others may help prevent the disease from starting, but in the highly oxidizing conditions of an established plaque, they may be futile—like trying to put out a bonfire with a water pistol.

The main exception to this generalization is vitamin C, taken under the condition known as dynamic flow. This high-dose, high-frequency procedure, which will be explained later in the book, can provide almost unlimited antioxidant protection.[81] Plaques are in an oxidized state that could, in principle, be reversed by bathing them in sufficient vitamin C.[82] Under dynamic flow conditions, vitamin C could enter the plaque in large enough amounts to act as an effective antioxidant. This implies that atherosclerosis may simply be a form of chronic scurvy.

IMPORTANT POINTS

- Some basic research in heart disease is being disregarded.

- Supplements such as arginine and chondroitin may prevent cardiovascular disease.

- Abnormal oxidation drives coronary disease.

- Suitable antioxidants could prevent cardiovascular disease.

- Sufficient powerful antioxidants might provide a cure.

- Atherosclerosis, coronary heart disease, and stroke could be manifestations of scurvy (vitamin C deficiency).

CHAPTER 8

QUENCHING
THE FIRE

*"Most ignorance is vincible ignorance.
We don't know because we don't want to know."*
—ALDOUS HUXLEY (1894–1963), *COLLECTED ESSAYS*

Atherosclerosis is notoriously hard to treat; one reason for this could be the difficulty of getting drugs or nutrients into the affected tissue. Not all anti-inflammatory agents will enter the plaque in high concentrations. Similarly, dietary antioxidants need to be able to enter the plaque if they are to be effective; once inside, they will lose electrons to free radicals. When an antioxidant has given up its electrons, it needs to leave the plaque or to be refreshed. This is the dilemma—the used antioxidant needs another antioxidant to reactivate it.

In healthy cells, antioxidants can be refreshed by the cells' metabolism, which provides additional antioxidant electrons. Cells burn food by oxidation to meet two continuous needs: energy and antioxidants. In an inflamed tissue, however, the cells suffer damage and stress. Preventing and repairing the damage caused by free radicals and other toxins overwhelms the cells' normal biochemistry. The cells are thus unable to provide enough energy to refresh their antioxidants and subsequently suffer further free radical damage. The tissue becomes increasingly oxidizing, which promotes further inflammation. However, use of the right antioxidants could stabilize or reverse the disease.

In animal studies, antioxidants have been shown to prevent atherosclerosis. Substances such as the tocotrienols, probucol, butylated hydroxytoluene, quercetin, and alpha tocopherol can slow the development of the disease and prevent arterial damage.[1] Epidemiology and clinical trials provide suggestive evidence for the benefits of antioxidants in humans.[2] Inadaquate levels of the antioxidant supplement quercetin, for example, may be associated with increased death from heart attack.[3] In general, however, studies on people have tended to use low doses of inappropriate supplements and give correspondingly conflicting results.

THE FIVE-A-DAY RULE

The recommendation that we should eat five portions a day of fruits and vegetables is intended to increase our intake of antioxidants and phytochemicals. However, this guidance is misleading and promises more than it can deliver. Even when the five-a-day recommendation is increased to nine portions, there is confusion about what constitutes a portion—it seems to mean different things to different people. We were of the impression that a portion might be equivalent to one apple, perhaps 100–200 grams. However, when we suggested this to a medical school professor, he said that could not be right, as people would have to eat one or two pounds of fruit and vegetables a day. According to the U.K. National Health Service, an average portion is 80 grams, which means five portions are equivalent to about 14 ounces a day and nine portions would be 24 ounces, or 1.5 pounds, a day.

Regardless of which portion size you consider, the biggest problem with the five-a-day recommendation is that this intake is not enough to provide sufficient antioxidants to compensate for our sugar-rich modern diet of fast foods and abnormal fats. Furthermore, the fruit may be blended into a smoothie, releasing large amounts of fructose. It is not clear if the potential harm of such a rapid influx of sugar is balanced by the benefits of released nutrients. Despite this, a smoothie might count as one or two of the required portions.

Similarly, the recommended vegetables could be raw or cooked. Cooking some vegetables may destroy their vitamin C; conversely others, including carrots, may provide more nutrients when cooked. Over the last half century, vegetables have become less rich in nutrients through changes in variety, farming, storage, and preservation methods.[4] Many reporters have noted the decline in taste and flavor, but the media has largely ignored the loss of nutrients. Vegetarians may be at lower risk from deficiency, but they can still have heart attacks.

The five-a-day initiative will not prevent you from having a heart attack or stroke. Superficially, the idea to eat more fruit and vegetables is an excellent recommendation for good health. Eating nutritious vegetables is good advice. However, the recommendation is aimed at getting us to obtain vitamins and nutrients from food, and the same authorities argue specifically against supplements. The vitamins, minerals, and other nutrients in five helpings of fruit and vegetables are unlikely to be sufficient to prevent or treat cardiovascular disease.

ARE VITAMINS A WASTE OF MONEY?

Corporate medicine typically scorns the benefits of vitamin supplements. A standard argument is that vitamins in food are beneficial to health, whereas those in supplements are not effective for protecting against disease. In some cases, this is an accurate statement, as some low-cost supplements contain synthetic vitamins. A classic example is vitamin E: poor-quality vitamin E supplements contain synthetic dl-alpha-tocopherol, whereas the natural molecule is pure d-alpha-tocopherol. Natural d-alpha-tocopherol is more biologically active than the synthetic dl-type. Moreover, high-quality vitamin E supplements contain several different forms of tocopherols and may also include tocotrienols. When clinical trials are performed by corporate medicine to test the value of vitamin E, however, researchers typically study an ineffective synthetic form, which would minimize any expected benefit.

Let us explain the difference between the two types of vitamin E. Organic molecules can exist in two forms, called optical isomers—the d-form and the l-form. They have an identical chemical formula and contain the same number of atoms, which are linked together in the same sequence. The difference between them is like that between our left and right hands: identical, but mirror images of each other. For ordinary chemical reactions, the two forms are indistinguishable. The exception is in biology.

Often, in the body, only one optical isomer can be used; this is because the enzymes needed for the biochemical reactions only act on one very precise molecular shape. Just as the right hand will not fit neatly into a left-handed glove, you generally need the correct optical isomer of a substance to fit an enzyme. The d- and l-forms of alpha-tocopherol thus do not have the same biological activity.[5] Moreover, synthetic l-alpha-tocopherol is so similar to the d-form that it might interfere with some biological reactions. By analogy, you could squeeze your right hand into a left-handed glove, but it would probably restrict your movement somewhat.

A study by the prestigious U.K. Heart Protection Study Collaborative Group of researchers and hospitals illustrates the problem. This large-scale study claimed boldly that antioxidant vitamins are not beneficial for heart disease.[6] The results were highlighted on television and splashed across the front pages of newspapers, with reports suggesting that antioxidant vitamins are a waste of money. However, the trial was not what it appeared; it was actually a comparison of low levels of antioxidants with a statin drug, and it had clear commercial implications for drug companies.

Patients were randomly allocated either to a treatment group given a combination of vitamin E (600 milligrams), vitamin C (250 milligrams), and beta-carotene (20 milligrams) daily or to a control group given a placebo. The supplements doubled blood levels of vitamin E, increased vitamin C by a third, and quadrupled levels of beta-carotene. Because the vitamin supplements did not alter the number of deaths, heart attacks, or strokes, the researchers concluded that the supplements provided no benefit.

The widely reported and highly generalized conclusion—that antioxidant vitamin supplementation was not effective—was unjustified. This five-year study did not include a wide enough range of antioxidant supplements to support such a sweeping generalization. In addition, the data presented did not support such a claim. Although the study cost well over $20 million and involved more than 20,000 adults between the ages of forty and eighty years, these subjects had coronary disease, other occlusive arterial disease, or diabetes. So, the study involved treatment of pre-existing disease, not prevention. The doses needed for treatment are much higher than those required for prevention.

Statins or Antioxidants?

Corporate medicine does not spend millions of dollars funding large-scale studies on vitamins that offer no potential for financial gain. In the Heart Protection Group study, additional results were announced for simvastatin, a cholesterol-lowering statin drug. It was claimed that adding simvastatin to the treatment of high-risk patients was beneficial, regardless of their blood cholesterol levels. Although the statin drug was reported to be safe, side effects are now becoming apparent, including heart failure, cancer, Parkinson's disease, and cataracts.[7]

The depletion of coenzyme Q_{10} caused by statins could result in heart failure and other muscle problems in some patients. The drug companies are aware of these issues; some have already taken out patents on combinations of statin drugs with nutritional supplements, such as CoQ_{10}[8] or the amino acid carnitine,[9] to prevent heart failure and other severe side effects. Presumably, CoQ_{10} will be added to their products when the side effects of the drugs have been fully established and have caused a public outcry. Dr. Julian Whitaker requested that the U.S. Food and Drug Administration

(FDA) recommend a warning label for statins, stating that CoQ_{10}, taken with these drugs, may help prevent damage to heart and other muscle in the longer term.[10]

The Heart Protection Group reported that 40 milligrams a day of simvastatin reduced heart attacks and strokes by about a quarter. Over a period of five years, they claimed that simvastatin could prevent 7–10 of every 100 high-risk people from suffering one of these major life-threatening events. Taken at face value, these benefits seem impressive—but they are misleading. Earlier, we described how the benefits of statin drugs were marginal for an individual. Even if the Heart Protection Group results were accurate, they relate only to the treatment of high-risk patients; the findings do not apply to the general population. Moreover, the results suggest that the benefit is unrelated to lowering high cholesterol levels.

Interestingly, there was little attempt to hide the study's economic implications. It was reported that if statins were used in clinical practice, the drug companies might benefit from billions of dollars worth of sales. The intended implications are clear: more people should be taking these profitable prescription drugs so the pharmaceutical companies will benefit from years of increased sales, while vitamin pills are a waste of money and should be thrown away.

A BAD EXPERIMENT

The Heart Protection Group study is biased and its conclusions are misleading. We have used it as an example of the poor design of clinical trials in nutrition and heart disease. Indeed, the experiment has many features we might include in a study, designed to draw the conclusion that vitamin supplements were ineffective or even harmful! Within the mantle of corporate medicine, honest researchers can be misled into wasting their time and research funds in an exercise that does little but confuse and deceive. Here are some of the problems.

Practically Unrepeatable

The size of the Heart Protection Group study makes it seem impressive, but restricts replication. The study extended over five years and, although this gives the appearance of scientific rigor, it increases the cost. Few doctors have the $20 million that would be necessary to repeat this work, even if they believe it to be biased. Replicating a study is the basis of science. Isaac Newton's law of gravitation is convincing—to test it, try dropping an apple; if it falls upward, Newton might have been mistaken. The ease with which a study can be repeated is an indication of its validity.

A Synthetic Vitamin

The Heart Protection Group results on vitamin E are biased. As mentioned previously, the study used the less biologically active synthetic vitamin E (dl-alpha-tocopherol). For a fair test, they would have used the natural mixed form, which is common in good-quality supplements. Instead, the Heart Protection Group's results applied only to their particular synthetic form of the supplement. It is not reasonable to use a substandard preparation and then suggest that the results apply generally to vitamin E. Unfortunately, this is not a new problem. For decades, negative studies on vitamin E have typically used the synthetic form.

The choice of synthetic vitamin E for the heart study would minimize any measured benefit. The synthetic vitamin E used in the statin study is biologically less effective than natural vitamin E. In addition, synthetic vitamin E is poorly absorbed, unless taken with a substantial amount of fat or oils. Supplementing pigs with natural vitamin E produces higher blood levels than if the synthetic form is used.[11] Furthermore, even if the researchers had used the natural form d-alpha-tocopherol, the results would not apply broadly to vitamin E, which consists of a number of chemical substances that possess the biological "vitamin E" activity. The various types of vitamin E have different properties. Alpha-tocopherol is generally considered a more powerful antioxidant than the other types. However, while in some circumstances alpha-tocopherol is a more potent antioxidant, gamma-tocopherol is linked more closely to protection against heart disease.[12] Gamma-tocopherol is also more common in the American diet.

Giving patients alpha-tocopherol might have had the unfortunate effect of lowering the availability of the more protective gamma-tocopherol. Gamma-tocopherol can exert a more powerful inhibitory effect on inflammation than alpha-tocopherol.[13] A Swedish study found that blood levels of gamma-tocopherol, but not alpha-tocopherol, were lower in patients with heart disease,[14] while the alpha-form was depleted in smokers.[15] Supplementing rats with alpha-tocopherol can decrease blood levels of gamma-tocopherol.[16] Many vitamin E tablets contain mixed combinations of the tocopherols, so the Heart Protection Group's decision to use only the alpha-form was misleading.

Synthetic vitamin E contains unnatural molecules that might make it less effective. These unnatural molecular forms have an S-shaped tail, with pronounced "kinks" that the natural forms do not have. While the synthetic vitamin E molecules with their twisted tails do enter membranes, they do not stay there. The kinked tails twist out of the plane of the membrane and prevent the molecules from stacking close together. Natural vitamin E molecules can pile together, like a set of spoons in a drawer, and are more suitable for acting as antioxidants in cell membranes. There are thus many reasons why a study based on synthetic substances provides little, if any, information on the benefits of natural antioxidants.

Nutrition or Pharmacology

A further cause for concern is that the Heart Protection Group used 600 milligrams (600 IU) of dl-alpha-tocopherol, biologically equivalent to about 400 IU d-alpha-tocopherol, which is too small a dose of vitamin E. If this was intended to be a study of the antioxidant effects of vitamin E, it failed before it started. Larger doses are needed in order for vitamin E to act as an antioxidant in the body. A minimum dose would be about 1,600 IU of natural vitamin E, and an even larger dose (3,200 IU) would be preferable.[17] The study was not testing a large enough dose of vitamin E to act as an antioxidant in a person with heart disease.

Additionally, if vitamin C is in short supply, vitamin E may itself become oxidized and then promote oxidation, acting as an oxidant instead of an antioxidant. This trial was a study of subjects with existing disease, so the dose given should have been larger than that necessary to prevent illness. The Heart Protection Group study confused normal nutrition for healthy individuals with pharmacology for treating patients who were already ill. Furthermore, the 250 milligrams of vitamin C used in the study was woefully inadequate. The claims for vitamin C supplements in preventing or treating cardiovascular disease are for much larger doses. By using only 250 milligrams, the trial used perhaps one-fiftieth of the effective intake of vitamin C.

The difference between nutritional and pharmacological doses was not noted by the media or corporate medicine. These basic errors were simply ignored.

Big Claims, Little Evidence

The Heart Protection Group study was unreliable and the results of this study are inapplicable. In our opinion, it would have been hard to design a more misleading experiment than this one, although the study was probably done in good faith. The doctors who conducted the study were presumably ethical and operated what they thought was a good, solid scientific investigation. However, performing good science is difficult and demanding. Designing an experiment takes thought, rather than slavishly following the cookbook methods of corporate medicine.

If we are hard on these researchers, it is because the Heart Protection Group made a strong and widely publicized claim, based on insufficient evidence. The researchers claimed their results showed antioxidant supplementation to be of no value. However, their study was useless—it did not apply to the dose, form, or nature of current supplements, or to the recognized health claims for their use.

CORRECTING MISTAKES

Researchers who study vitamins and heart disease sometimes seem set on avoiding the issue of benefit. One interesting study of vitamin supplements by Dr. Michael Gaziano and colleagues determined that they offered no benefit for people with coronary heart disease. This enormous study involved 83,639 subjects with no history of cardiovascular disease or cancer. Over the course of the study, which lasted five-and-a-half years, a total of 1,037 people died of cardiovascular disease, including 608 deaths from heart attack. The researchers stated, "In this large cohort of apparently healthy U.S. male physicians, self-selected supplementation with vitamin E, vitamin C, or multivitamins was not associated with a significant decrease in total cardiovascular disease or coronary heart disease mortality."[18] This statement was wrong.

A California doctor, Joel Simon, read the paper and noticed that the conclusion was false—one group of subjects had indicated that vitamins C and E provided a large and significant benefit.[19] The low-risk subjects, taking both vitamin C and vitamin E supplements, showed a 41 percent reduction in mortality from coronary heart disease and 34 percent reduction in mortality from cardiovascular disease. If these results were correct, 41 out of every 100 low-risk people who died of a heart attack might have lived had they taken supplements. These are large benefits but, strangely, the original researchers ignored their results! However, when the error was brought to light, Gaziano and colleagues admitted their mistake. They agreed with Joel Simon that their study results indicated a 28–41 percent reduction in mortality, with the greatest effect being in the subgroup taking both vitamins C and E.[20] So, rather than being of no benefit, the vitamins appeared to save lives.

The results that were missed related to people with low risk factors. Previous studies had also shown benefit in low-risk individuals taking supplements. This was in contrast to high-risk groups, which did not show the same effect. One possible explanation is that the low doses of supplements employed in these studies were sufficient to benefit those with healthier cardiovascular systems but were inadequate for people predisposed to the illness. In reply, Gaziano accurately explained that the results suggested that vitamins C and E are effective in the early stages of cardiovascular disease (CVD). In his words: "Many observational studies among those at usual or low-risk of CVD suggest a benefit of these vitamins. These findings from our study as well as the conflicting data from trials and observational studies raise the possibility that vitamins E and C are most effective in the earliest stages of atherosclerosis."

In the end, Dr. Gaziano's results were in line with those from earlier studies that had showed significant benefit. But although his research replicated previous observations, the positive findings were initially ignored, with the researchers suggesting that they could have been a chance result. This explanation is simply confused, as all statistical results are based on chance (probability). The result was statistically significant, which means the result should have been properly reported.

Here is a clear example of a single large experiment being misunderstood by the researchers who conducted it. Fortunately, the error was caught and the researchers were then able to correct their bias and explain the position more accurately. However, the observation that a group of scientists can be so easily misled into misreporting the benefits of vitamins is sobering.

IMPORTANT POINTS

- Oxidation and free radical damage drive atherosclerosis.

- Antioxidants may be used to prevent or treat heart disease.

- Most antioxidants are insufficiently powerful to reverse the disease.

- Five servings of fruit and vegetables are no substitute for nutritional supplements.

- Trials of antioxidants are often misleading.

CHAPTER 9

AN INFECTIOUS
DISEASE?

*"People who have chronic infections—and gum
disease is one of the major chronic infections—
are at increased risk later in life for atherosclerosis
and coronary heart disease."*
—RICHARD STEIN, M.D.

For years, the role of infection in common illnesses such as heart
disease and stomach ulcers has been downplayed. Researchers
claimed that heart attack and stroke are not caused by infection—
people do not "catch" heart attacks, as they might a common cold.
Rather, heart attacks are said to be the result of multiple risk factors associated with lifestyle. Similarly, stomach ulcers have been
attributed to numerous risk factors, such as spicy food, emotional stress, or type A personality.

In 1982, however, Dr. Barry Marshall and Dr. Robin Warren
found a bacterium called *Helicobacter pylori* in the stomachs of
people suffering with gastritis and stomach ulcers. They went on
to show that such ulcers are often the result of bacterial infection.
Corporate medicine initially downplayed this finding and delayed
funding for clinical trials. The critics assumed that bacteria could
not survive the stomach's acidity, which is about as corrosive as
the fluid in a car battery. Furthermore, Marshall and Warren's
work did not agree with years of research on the risk factors for

peptic ulcers; it also threatened to destroy the market for some highly profitable drugs. Their findings were eventually recognized over twenty years later, when Marshall and Warren were awarded the 2005 Nobel Prize in Medicine.

As a result of the finding that ulcers arise from an infectious disease, we might expect serious consideration to be given to the notion that other common long-term diseases could be caused by infections.[1] It is no longer realistic to suggest that heart attack could not possibly be caused in this way. Currently, the evidence suggests that any infection linked to heart disease is more likely to be opportunistic than causative.[2] The cause of chronic inflammation of the arteries is persistent oxidation, free radical damage, and mechanical injury. Nevertheless, when inflammation and tissue damage are present, chronic infection may take hold, and, once established, it encourages further inflammation.

In this chapter, we look at how bacteria and viruses can complicate our understanding of cardiovascular disease. Research in this area has been restricted by a lack of resources; funds have presumably been consumed by cholesterol research. As a result, our account is a brief description of some of the main bacteria that could be implicated in heart disease, with an overview of the mechanisms involved. The main thought to take from this chapter is that cardiovascular disease could have an infectious element. The assumption that infection is not involved in heart disease is another example of the shortsightedness of corporate medicine.

The idea that heart disease might be an infection was suggested in the early twentieth century and is now being reconsidered, because risk factors do not fully explain the development of the disease.[3] Many people who suffer a heart attack or occlusive stroke do not have the "traditional" risk factors.[4] More importantly, the hypothesis that heart disease arises from an infection implies that an effective immune system is essential for good cardiovascular health and freedom from atherosclerosis. This opens up a range of potential approaches to prevention and treatment.

In the past, it was assumed that the healthy human body was

internally sterile and that blood and tissues were aseptic and free from microorganisms. People thought our immune systems were constantly on patrol and prevented all infection in healthy individuals. However, we now know that even healthy people can have bacteria and viruses in their bloodstream and tissues. The assumption that the body tissues are sterile may remind the reader of the blinkered outlook on ulcers: a result of the belief that the human stomach was sterile.

A number of infectious agents might contribute to heart disease. Many of them are common infections, though they carry the usual long medical names. They include influenzas A and B, adenovirus, enterovirus, Coxsackie B4 virus, and various herpes viruses, especially cytomegalovirus. Both viruses and bacteria seem to be implicated. We cannot avoid the jargon of the names. Fortunately, the particular types of bugs are not our main concern, it is more important to appreciate that a range of organisms may infect inflamed arteries.

Microorganisms can colonize arterial plaques. Viruses are known to infect the cells of blood vessels,[5] and atherosclerotic patches may be more available to viral attack.[6] Bacterial infections may also be involved.[7] In particular, the bacteria found in common gum infections (gingivitis) are associated with cardiovascular disease. Multiple disease organisms are implicated, and the infection could provide a trigger for clot formation,[8] heart attack, and stroke. The particular microorganism that infects a plaque may be unimportant; it could simply be a matter of which one happens to exploit the damage in the arterial wall.

The diversity of microorganisms found in plaques may reflect such opportunistic infection, as a damaged artery is an opportunity awaiting colonization. Furthermore, multiple organisms could act together to increase inflammation.[9] In the case of heart disease, it appears unlikely that a single infectious agent is causative, as was the case with stomach ulcers.[10] The available evidence suggests that the overall microbial burden on the patient is linked to opportunistic infection of the arteries.[11] However, the likelihood that a septic plaque was not started by the bacteria is little comfort to a person about to suffer a cardiac event.

Infection feeds the fire of inflammation and oxidation, aggravating the atherosclerosis. Viral and other infections can increase free-radical damage.[12] Even the occasionally reported absence of an identified microbe does not imply that such organisms do not usually play a central part in the process.[13] If an infection produces or contributes to chronic local inflammation, it may cause a minor irritation to become a dangerously active arterial plaque.

In animal models of atherosclerosis, both viral and bacterial infections can aggravate lesions. Many such pathogens may accelerate atherosclerosis.[14] Recent data suggest that the greater the number of separate organisms that afflict an individual, the greater is the risk of developing atherosclerosis. This risk also reflects levels of variability in host susceptibility to the pathogens. People at greatest risk are those who are not able to generate a strong immune response and whose bodies are not able to control inflammation. The next few sections detail some of the organisms that are believed to be involved in cardiovascular disease.

VIRAL INFECTION

Herpes virus is a well-known cause of unpleasant human infections. This class of virus will infect other animals and has thus been described as somewhat promiscuous. In animals, herpes can cause atherosclerosis; this finding supports the idea that heart disease could be infectious and brings the cholesterol hypothesis into question. Marek's disease is a highly contagious herpes infection that affects poultry, causing weight loss, paralysis, and tumors. In the 1970s, researchers found that the Marek virus could lead to development of atherosclerosis in chickens.[15]

The infected chickens developed fibrous atherosclerotic changes, rather like those found in the human illness.[16] Striking plaques were seen in the large coronary arteries of chickens with both normal and high cholesterol levels. These plaques had a similar discrete distribution and appearance to those in humans. By contrast, chickens that were not infected with the Marek virus did not develop large plaques, regardless of whether or not they were fed high-cholesterol diets. These results suggest viral infection can cause cardiovascular disease.

The infective nature of Marek's disease does not mean that the virus definitely causes the illness directly. The involvement of viruses in the progression of the disease in birds may be indirect; for example, the virus could stimulate the immune system, generating a local inflammatory response.[17] Notably, the development of atherosclerosis in these chickens might be prevented by immunization against herpes.[18] By analogy, using nutritional supplements to strengthen immunity in humans could protect against heart attack and stroke.

Inspired by finding the viral connection in chickens, researchers investigated human herpes. Herpes viruses are common in humans and cause widespread, long-term infections and diseases, including cold sores, chickenpox, shingles, Kaposi's sarcoma, and glandular fever (also known as infectious mononucleosis or the kissing disease). For example, cytomegalovirus, a form of herpes, is prevalent in the human population and can cause inflammation of the eye (retinitis) and an infection similar to mononucleosis. The proportion of people in the population infected with cytomegalovirus increases with age and the majority are infected by the time they reach old age.[19] Atherosclerosis might eventually be added to this list of herpes-related illnesses.

By the 1980s, scientists were beginning to take the idea of atherosclerosis as an infectious disease seriously. They already knew that atherosclerosis in chickens could be caused by infection.[20] The atherosclerotic plaques in Japanese quail were examined and signs of herpes infection (Marek virus DNA) were consistently found in the embryos that were genetically vulnerable; far fewer of the unsusceptible quail embryos had the virus.[21] These disturbing results suggest that atherosclerosis, in birds at least, may be linked to viral infection passed down the generations.

Of course, it is possible that the disease in birds might be specific to those animals and have no connection to human illness. However, later research demonstrated that rats infected with the herpes virus developed blood vessel lesions,[22] and mice with herpes are also susceptible to atherosclerosis.[23] As mammals, the physiology of rats and mice is closer to that of humans than is that of birds. Further circumstantial evidence was discovered when plaques in humans were examined for herpes simplex and viral DNA was found.[24] DNA from other herpes viruses has also been found in humans, within arteries and in association with atherosclerotic plaques.[25] Cytomegalovirus, a herpes virus that can cause a form of glandular fever, may be linked to aortic aneurisms in humans.[26] So, experiments suggest that a virus could trigger human cardiovascular disease.

Clinical evidence also indicates that herpes may be implicated in heart disease.[27] Coronary patients have an increased antibody response to cytomegalovirus.[28] Diabetics display both an impaired immune response and a greatly increased tendency for cardiovascular disease. Moreover, antibodies for the virus may be higher in diabetics with arterial disease.[29] By 1995, active viruses had not been isolated from human atherosclerotic plaques,[30] but a decade later they were found and associated with specific cell types.[31] With time, the evidence linking infection to heart disease is increasing.

Viral infection does not necessarily cause an obvious illness. Some viruses can hide within cells. A latent virus can lie dormant for years, until the immune system weakens and is unable to keep it in check. Latent herpes is common, especially in patients with atherosclerosis.[32] The smooth muscle cells in arteries and the white blood cells that are attracted to sites of arterial damage may each harbor the virus.[33] Since immunosuppression would be predicted to promote the viral growth, patients with latent infections would be prone to atherosclerosis.

Transplant patients are at particular risk of infections, partly because of their use of immunosuppressive drugs. In heart transplant patients, viral infection is associated with reduced long-term survival.[34] Infection in heart recipients is associated with more frequent rejection, graft atherosclerosis, and death. In immunosuppressed transplant patients, there is an increased incidence of herpes infection and a greater frequency of rejection, together with accelerated atherosclerosis.[35] Transplanted blood vessels are at particular risk. Patients who are infected with herpes are more likely to die from cardiovascular disease in the transplanted heart.[36] High levels of herpes antibodies are found preferentially in the blood of transplant patients who suffer atherosclerosis.[37] Additionally, the graft loss rate is greater. Mechanical stress and infection can combine to thwart the surgeon's efforts to save the patient's life.

As described earlier, transplant patients can suffer very rapid atherosclerosis. Even children can be affected. Since the patients are immunosuppressed, it immediately suggests the idea that infection may be the problem. Heart transplant patients infected with cytomegalovirus are particularly prone to the illness,[38] and atherosclerosis is a major cause of late-occurring graft failure and subsequent death.[39] Transplant atherosclerosis differs from the traditional disease, in that it is more diffuse and calcification is rare.[40] Also, the disease progresses rapidly.

Earlier, we explained how transplants cause mechanical stress in blood vessels. The blood vessels are damaged by surgery, and connections between vessels of different sizes may be necessary, corresponding to the dimensions of the new organ. These connections disturb blood flow and form sites of increased arterial stress and scar tissue. Arterial damage, abnormal blood flow, and immunosuppression combine to create local conditions favorable to the development of inflammation and infection. The consequence may be failure of the transplanted organ. Re-transplantation is a common response to transplant atherosclerosis, though it is not highly effective. Rapid atherosclerosis can soon develop again in the second transplanted organ.

Atherosclerosis, heart attack, and stroke are typically considered adult diseases, occurring particularly in elderly people. They can occur in younger adults but the frequency is much lower. Most of the established risk factors, such as high cholesterol, are built on this premise. However, atherosclerosis can be relatively rapid in onset and can sometimes occur in the very young. Even in children, heart transplants often fail as a result of atherosclerotic changes;[41] this finding is inconsistent with the idea that lifestyle risk factors play a primary role. Conversely, the disease in these children is easily explained by inflammation and oxidation, which may precipitate infection.

These results illustrate how viral infection may be involved in the progression of the disease. Periodically activated virus may have a role in the pathogenesis of atherosclerosis. When the arteries of young trauma victims were examined, herpes virus was found both in normal sections of artery and in early atherosclerotic lesions.[42] Herpes-infected people may be at higher risk of atherosclerosis.

Understanding the role of infection may give rise to new treatments. Since herpes viruses have been implicated in the initiation and development of atherosclerosis,[43] immunization against these might prevent the disease.[44] However, this suggestion overlooks the role of other infectious agents. Immunization is specific to a single virus and is unlikely to be effective. The herpes virus is not the only infective organism and a nonspecific anti-infective agent would be more appropriate. Perhaps the ideal course would be to maintain a strong immune system.

Herpes, like other viral infections, involves oxidation and free-radical damage.[45] Antioxidant supplements may support the immune system and protect against free radicals. Some antioxidants, such as vitamin C, can prevent viral replication. It is even possible that aspirin acts as an antioxidant when used in atherosclerotic patients, which could also inhibit herpes replication.[46] Cytomegalovirus damages coronary arteries by a progressive inflammatory response that involves proliferation of smooth muscle cells. Antioxidants can inhibit this cell proliferation.[47] Notably, transplant patients with chronic graft damage have been found to be deficient in the antioxidant mineral selenium.[48] Supplementation with selenium and other antioxidants would be a wise precaution for all those at high risk of cardiovascular disease.

AIDS patients provide another clue that the immune system protects against heart disease. The human immunodeficiency virus (HIV), which is implicated in the development of AIDS, is associated with suppression of the immune response. Patients infected with HIV display an increased rate of development of atherosclerosis.[49] The resulting arterial lesions are intermediate in structure between normal plaque and transplant disease. There is a pattern consistent with viral infection; however, the main risk may come from bacteria and from *Chlamydia* in particular.

CHLAMYDIA

Most people have heard of chlamydia as a common form of sexually transmitted disease. Many people infected with the *C. trachomatis* bacteria have no symptoms and may be unaware that they have the disease. If untreated, however, sexually transmitted chlamydial infection can cause serious illness. In many parts of the world, it is a common but preventable cause of blindness. Like the infection, the damage that chlamydia causes is often unnoticed. In about 40 percent of women, untreated infection spreads into the uterus or fallopian tubes, causing pelvic inflammatory disease (PID). This can result in permanent harm to the uterus, fallopian tubes, and surrounding tissues. Ultimately the damage can cause chronic pelvic pain, infertility, and increased risk of ectopic pregnancy, in which a fetus develops outside the womb. In men, complications are less common but occasionally the infection spreads to the epididymis, the tube that carries sperm from the testis, causing pain and sometimes sterility.

In connection with heart disease, however, we are mainly concerned with another form of chlamydia, called *Chlamydophila pneumoniae*, which was isolated relatively recently. This species was not found until the 1960s because of the difficulty in isolating and culturing these bacteria.[50] C. pneumoniae is transmitted from person to person in the air, and all ages are at risk of infection, though it is most common in school-age children. By age twenty, about half of all adults in the United States show evidence of infection. In adults, researchers have estimated that C. pneumoniae causes about 10 percent of all community-acquired pneumonia, and 5 percent of bronchitis and sinusitis, although most infections do not produce symptoms. Despite this relatively benign nature, infections can flare up, causing common and important respiratory tract diseases, and re-infection remains common throughout life.

The association of heart disease with Chlamydia appears to be based solidly on the available evidence.[51] Indeed, it may be the most important infectious agent in atherosclerosis.[52] In young adults, this organism is more frequently found in association with plaques than in normal arterial wall.[53] There is some evidence for antibodies in the blood early in the development of atherosclerosis.[54] Some researchers have reported that infection with Chlamydia[55] may be a greater risk than with Helicobacter or herpes viruses,[56] and evidence for Chlamydia's involvement in cardiovascular disease is stronger.[57] Although the accumulating data is convincing,[58] this does not indicate that it is a cause of the disease.[59] Studies of antibodies in blood provide only circumstantial evidence; both the infection and the atherosclerosis could be secondary to something else—a weakened immune system, for example. A preliminary study on the use of antibiotics in atherosclerotic patients with C. pneumoniae suggested a decrease in acute coronary events after one month.[60] However, although some antibiotic intervention studies have shown benefits, a number of negative studies have also emerged.

While the association of Chlamydia with atherosclerosis appears to have been established, it is not clear whether it is causative or is an opportunistic infection. The infection thrives with a depressed immune system and increases inflammation. As with any infection, damaged tissue increases the opportunity for chlamydial growth.

GUM DISEASE

One particular source of bacterial infection may be a constant threat to the bloodstream. Gum disease is a potential source of infection as bacteria are released into the blood, searching for a new tissue to invade.

It may seem hard to believe, but brushing your teeth regularly and taking care of your basic dental hygiene may help you avoid a heart attack in the long run. Several bacteria normally found in diseased gums have been found in arterial plaque.[61] Infected gums present a range of microorganisms to the bloodstream, and damaged arteries are easy targets for such infections. A damaged arterial wall could be as inviting as a gum to opportunistic bacteria. At this point, the importance of dental hygiene in relation to cardiovascular disease is not clear, as studies have produced conflicting results.[62] Gingivitis may increase the risk of atherosclerosis slightly.[63] This limited effect suggests that gum disease is just an additional source of infection for the colonization of inflamed arteries. Nevertheless, good dental hygiene is a simple self-help option for people with cardiovascular disease.

INFECTION AND ATHEROSCLEROSIS

While it might not produce the initial lesion,[64] chronic infection appears to promote the development of atherosclerosis, as it accelerates the development of plaque by promoting local inflammation. The resulting inflammation is probably not specific to a particular disease-causing organism.[65] Any area of damage is an opportunity for colonization by a microorganism. The role of the microorganism may be to infect, grow, and cause plaques to rupture more quickly than would otherwise be the case.

If a bacterial infection is responsible for causing atherosclerosis, suitable antibiotics should prevent or even be an effective treatment for the disease.[66] An alternative approach for corporate medicine might be vaccination.[67] In the late 1990s, two pilot studies using antibiotics appeared to improve the outlook for coronary artery disease.[68] Of course, antibiotics only work against susceptible bacteria and are completely ineffective against viruses. Antiviral drug therapy—such as that used to treat herpes infections in transplant patients[69]—has also been proposed,[70] though resistance can develop rapidly.[71] Thus, the prospects for both antibiotic and antiviral therapies appear limited. Even if effective, these two approaches are likely to help only a small proportion of patients.

Active infection often involves a compromised immune system.[72] As they age, people who have strong immune systems may have a distinct advantage in avoiding the ravages of atherosclerosis, heart disease, and stroke. One way of achieving a robust immune system is through good nutrition. Improved nutrition has long been associated with increasing life expectancy and resistance to disease. The role of vitamin D in supporting the immune system is increasingly recognized and deficiency is associated with compromised immunity.[73] Supplements may be essential, particularly vitamins C and D_3.

IMPORTANT POINTS

- Heart disease and strokes could be triggered or aggravated by infectious diseases.

- Deaths from infections have fallen greatly in modern times, mainly due to improved nutrition.

- Current nutritional deficiencies and other risk factors can exacerbate chronic infections.

- Boosting the immune system may help prevent cardiovascular disease.

CHAPTER 10

LINUS PAULING
AND VITAMIN C

"Facts do not cease to exist because they are ignored."
—ALDOUS HUXLEY

Several independent scientists and doctors, including renowned Nobel Prize-winning chemist Linus Pauling, have concluded that heart disease is a symptom of scurvy. Scurvy is caused by vitamin C deficiency and, in the olden days, it was a disease greatly feared by seamen who spent long periods at sea. Symptoms of scurvy include disruption of the immune system, shortage of the structural protein collagen, and bleeding from the mucous membranes. The deficiency will ultimately result in death, if it is not corrected.

Pauling was famous for being ahead of his time, and his scientific foresight led to breakthroughs in several disciplines. However, in the cautionary words of Albert Szent-Györgyi, the Nobel laureate who discovered vitamin C: "It is fine to be one step ahead of everyone else—just don't be two steps ahead." He elaborated, "If everybody says that you are wrong, then you are one step ahead. But there is one situation which is better still, when everyone begins to laugh about you, then you know you are two steps ahead." With vitamin C, Pauling may have been three steps ahead of most scientists working in the field.

Linus Pauling is now famous (some would even say infamous) for his promotion of vitamin C. Pauling did not originate the theory that atherosclerosis is a form of scurvy—the idea was decades old when he became involved, and experimental evidence was already accumulating. However, he applied his intellect to the issue, before staking his reputation on his findings and those of earlier scientists, who had been ignored by the medical establishment. Despite this long history and the valiant efforts of Pauling and other pioneers, the action of high-dose vitamin C against heart disease has yet to be investigated clinically by corporate medicine.

One of the earliest researchers to link vitamin C deficiency and heart disease was Dr. J.C. Paterson, a Canadian pathologist. In the 1940s, Paterson proposed that shortage of vitamin C is a cause of atherosclerosis, heart attack, and stroke. Despite being a minority viewpoint, the idea has gradually gained experimental support. Work by other scientists also suggests that vitamin C deficiency can lead to atherosclerosis.[1]

Vitamin C can be linked to heart disease in several ways. High levels of sugar are known to inhibit the uptake of vitamin C into cells; thus, the increased atherosclerosis commonly found in diabetes could be a result of secondary scurvy. Researchers have noted that shortage of vitamin C disturbs cholesterol metabolism. It also increases histamine levels, which can damage the lining of the arteries, leading to atherosclerosis. By 1976, clinical and experimental evidence that chronic vitamin C deficiency leads to the abnormal accumulation of cholesterol in tissues of the body—and to atherosclerosis in particular—was growing.[2]

ANIMALS RARELY HAVE HEART ATTACKS

As mentioned, animals do not usually suffer from coronary heart disease; the illness is rare in both carnivores and herbivores. Humans are distinctly susceptible, which suggests that something about human biochemistry is different from that of most other animals. An outstanding biochemical difference is that, as we evolved, humans lost the ability to synthesize vitamin C. Most comparable animals manufacture vitamin C internally, in large amounts. Interestingly, guinea pigs also depend on dietary vitamin C, and like humans are susceptible to a form of atherosclerosis, if their intake is insufficient. Guinea pigs with vitamin C deficiency have been shown to form plaques, regardless of the presence of cholesterol in their diet.

In contrast, dogs synthesize vitamin C internally, producing the daily equivalent of about 2.5 grams in a human. Yet, despite eating a meat-based diet containing potentially large amounts of saturated fat and cholesterol, dogs rarely have heart attacks. In a study of 3,022 x-rays from dogs, only nineteen showed coronary mineralization, which is a sign of advanced atherosclerosis.[3] Nevertheless, some may not synthesize all the vitamin C that they require. Selective breeding could result in particular domestic dogs, such as the German Shepherd (Alsatian), having a vitamin C deficiency. Certain breeds also suffer a form of congenital hip dysplasia that may be corrected with supplemental vitamin C.[4] The relatively rare cases in which dogs develop atherosclerosis may be associated with diabetes. Alternatively, infection with *Chlamydia* may be involved.[5] In the x-ray study mentioned above, 671 cats were also imaged and not one showed mineralization. However, feeding domestic cats an abnormally high-fat diet for several months can produce signs of atherosclerosis.[6]

Other animals that manufacture their own vitamin C internally are resistant to atherosclerosis. However, pigs have been used as an experimental model for atherosclerosis—research suggests that if pigs are fed a high-fat diet, they can develop a form of the disease. In particular, diabetic pigs, which are relatively short of vitamin C, can get atherosclerosis.[7] However, unlike those in humans, pig plaques do not usually develop their own blood supply or microvessels, nor do they rupture in the same way.[8] Birds have varied requirements for vitamin C intake and the available data is sparse. Some, like humans, are dependent on their diet whilst others can make it internally.[9] Certain birds, such as old parrots or cockatoos, can become atherosclerotic.[10]

Wild baboons, which like humans and other primates do not

manufacture their own vitamin C, get a form of atherosclerosis, though they do not make good animal models of the disease.[11] Similarly, monkeys in the wild may develop arterial lesions,[12] which may become worse in captivity if they are fed a high-cholesterol diet.[13] However, the atherosclerosis observed in most mammals is milder than the human disease.[14] Some animals, such as goats, have higher levels of vitamin C than domestic dogs[15] and may boost production when stressed. This stress related increase is large; it has been estimated to be equivalent to a human going from 13 to 100 grams per day. Bears and squirels increase their vitamin C levels during hibernation.[16] A high-cholesterol diet need not induce arterial oxidation in rats, which can synthesize vitamin C. However, a similar diet produces damaging oxidation in the quail, a bird that is susceptible to arterial plaque formation[17] and may require dietary vitamin C.

Linus Pauling read the scientific literature on vitamin C and became convinced that high levels protect animals from heart attacks. He suggested that the government recommendations for human intake would leave people deficient, as the blood levels in people would be far lower than those generally found in animals. Animals are resistant to the development of atherosclerosis, and when the illness does occur, it is far less likely to produce heart attack than in people. The observation that cardiovascular disease is closely associated with the inability to synthesize vitamin C is powerful suggestive evidence for the cause of the disease. Shortage of vitamin C provides a simple and consistent explanation of why people die of heart disease and stroke.

ACTIVE PLAQUES

Vitamin C is necessary for maintaining artery strength and plaque integrity, making plaques less liable to rupture.[18] Plaque itself is rarely a problem—most damage is caused by blood clots that form as the plaque ruptures. Vitamin C deficiency weakens plaques, leaving them susceptible to mechanical injury and increasing the likelihood of clot formation.[19]

Based on these findings, Pauling suggested that atherosclerosis is dangerous when the plaque becomes unstable through shortage of vitamin C. Experimental evidence supports this idea. In a strain of mice that do not synthesize vitamin C or LDL cholesterol, the plaques contain less collagen and are more likely to rupture than those found in normal mice.[20] The researchers found these fragile plaques could be stabilized by supplementing with vitamin C, although this did not alter the number of plaques that the mice developed.

The idea of stabilizing plaques to prevent heart attacks is not new. In the 1940s, Paterson observed that strokes started with the formation of blood clots in arterial plaques.[21] Microscopic examination suggested to Paterson that the clots developed from damage to the capillaries in a plaque. When these clots broke away, they became lodged in blood vessels in the brain and caused a stroke. As a result of his findings, Paterson suggested that high blood pressure stresses the blood vessels and damages capillaries.[22] In so doing, he described a mechanism of action by which high blood pressure could produce a stroke or heart attack. Since fragile capillaries are a sign of scurvy, Paterson reasoned that heart attacks and strokes may be caused by vitamin C deficiency.

If vitamin C deficiency causes heart attacks, people who have scurvy would be particularly at risk. Sir Hans Krebs, another eminent Nobel Prize winner, tested this hypothesis in an infamous study of scurvy in Sheffield, England.[23] The research was conducted during the World War II and the subjects were conscientious objectors: people who were morally opposed to warfare and volunteered for the experiments as an alternative to military service. In 1996, the experiment was reviewed at the Nuremberg doctor trials, because of the supposed death of one of its subjects.[24] The project, however, was deemed ethical.

In Krebs' experiment, ten volunteers were deprived of vitamin C and all developed scurvy, though none died during the clinical trial. Two subjects (20 percent) showed symptoms of heart attack, which subsided when they were given vitamin C. This study provides direct clinical confirmation of the animal research that links scurvy to heart attack. Despite the study being considered ethical at the time, deliberately inducing scurvy in humans is an experiment that is unlikely to be repeated. We have been given a warning that scurvy might induce heart attack and that such trials are dangerous. However, the implication of this small trial—that scurvy causes heart attack—seems to have been forgotten.

FURTHER STUDIES ON VITAMIN C

By the early 1950s, Dr. C.G. Willis became interested in the causes of atherosclerosis.[25] Following Paterson's lead, Willis surmised that if animals were deprived of vitamin C, they would get atherosclerosis. In retrospect, this seems to be an obvious experiment, considering the results of Paterson's research and the heart attacks produced in humans during the Sheffield experiment. The first problem was to select a suitable animal. Most animals make their own vitamin C and do not need it in the diet, so Willis turned to the classic experimental animal, the guinea pig.

Guinea pigs have been used in scientific experiments since the 1600s. Like humans, guinea pigs require vitamin C from the diet and are thus suitable for basic experimentation. This made them particularly useful for experiments into vitamin C and scurvy, early in the twentieth century. Guinea pigs became popular experimental animals because of their relatively low upkeep costs and the similarity of their physiology to that of humans—particularly their requirement for vitamin C. Indeed, the convenience of guinea pigs in the early studies of infectious diseases may have been because of their need for dietary vitamin C: the animal's immune system does not function well without high levels of the vitamin. Their resultant sensitivity to infection was important during early medical research into the cause of tuberculosis. In 1882, Dr. Robert Koch, the "father of bacteriology," used guinea pigs to show that

Mycobacterium tuberculosis causes tuberculosis.[26] The experiment would have been unsuccessful with most other small animals, but Koch realized that guinea pigs were particularly suitable, because of their susceptibility to infections.[27]

Papers on vitamin C from the 1930s, when the substance was isolated, reveal that the intake needed for good health in humans was already considered controversial. In guinea pigs, a low intake was found to prevent scurvy, although higher doses were apparently quite safe. Scurvy was a major concern of these early researchers, who assumed that a minimum intake—sufficient to prevent the acute symptoms of scurvy—would suffice for health. However, even at this early stage, experiments were beginning to show increased vulnerability to illness in animals with low or inadequate intakes. Rather strangely, it was assumed that humans needed only the minimum amount to prevent acute scurvy, whereas zoo animals and pets were often given far more, to ensure good health!

Standard vitamin C intake recommendations for guinea pigs range from 6 milligrams per day for an adult to 20 milligrams per day for a pregnant female.[28] This would be the equivalent to 1.4 grams a day for a 70-kg (150-pound) human adult, or 4.6 grams during pregnancy. In other words, these recommendations for guinea pigs are far higher than the government's Recommended Dietary Allowance (RDA) values for people, which are in the region of 100 mg per day. The recommendations for guinea pigs are consistent with the gram-level range suggested by Linus Pauling for humans; his initial suggestion was for an intake of 1 gram, though he increased this recommendation with time and, by the time of his death, he was consuming 18 grams a day.

To test the idea that atherosclerosis is a form of scurvy, Willis fed 145 guinea pigs a diet high in cholesterol, together with varying amounts of vitamin C. Guinea pigs are generally vegetarian and do not eat much cholesterol; consequently, in contrast to humans, these animals do not have good internal controls for cholesterol.[29] Furthermore, cholesterol in the guinea pigs' diet tends to be deposited throughout their body tissues, rather than in the arterial wall. Nevertheless, Willis' research showed that guinea pigs that were given low levels of vitamin C developed a form of atherosclerosis. In animals with vitamin C deficiency, high intakes of cholesterol resulted in plaques. However, vitamin C supplementation was found to lower the incidence of plaques, even when cholesterol intake was high. When injected, vitamin C prevented plaque formation in about half the animals that had overdosed on cholesterol. Furthermore, the plaques in guinea pigs that consumed high levels of both cholesterol and vitamin C were less severe than those in animals with vitamin C deficiency alone.

There has been ample research showing that guinea pigs develop atherosclerosis when fed a diet low in vitamin C.[30] Pauling also experimented with three guinea pigs and confirmed that a low intake could induce atherosclerosis.[31] Further research has shown that guinea pigs taking inadequate dietary vitamin C develop high blood cholesterol,[32] high blood lipids,[33] atherosclerosis,[34] and increased oxidative stress.[35] This raises the possibility that high cholesterol and blood lipids in people with atherosclerosis may simply be a marker for chronically poor nutrition.

A high-cholesterol diet with low vitamin C also produces atherosclerosis in guinea pigs.[36] However, the association between dietary cholesterol and tissue cholesterol found in guinea pigs does not occur in humans.[37] Humans are omnivorous and have become adapted to eating meat and animal fats. Despite this, the established relationship between low vitamin C and atherosclerosis in guinea pigs may reflect the cause of the human disease. This suggestion is supported by the Sheffield experiments discussed earlier, in which two of ten subjects with experimentally induced scurvy suffered heart attack symptoms.

Following his early research, Willis had confirmed that shortage of vitamin C could cause atherosclerosis in guinea pigs. His next question concerned whether increasing vitamin C intake might reverse the disease in other animals. He chose rabbits for these experiments, because it had already been established that feeding rabbits an unnaturally high cholesterol diet can lead the substance to be deposited in their arteries. Like guinea pigs, rabbits are herbivores, so a diet high in cholesterol is abnormal for them. They differ from guinea pigs in that they can synthesize their own vitamin C. However, rabbits may not produce as much of the vitamin as they need.[38] This is not surprising, as their usual vegetarian diet provides a high intake of the vitamin. Manufacturing vitamin C internally takes energy, which might be required for running—to escape a fox, for example. Thus, evolution would favor animals that use their food as a supplementary source of the vitamin, in order to save energy for basic survival.

Rabbits are clearly not ideal animals in which to study acute scurvy, though they may be appropriate for researching suboptimal intakes of vitamin C. Their requirement for vitamin C would increase under conditions of physiological stress. Laboratory animals can be stressed by their conditions and by their diet. Experimental rabbits are often fed chow pellets, which may not include vitamin C. A high-cholesterol diet with no dietary vitamin C is not healthy for rabbits and would be a source of physiological stress.

Willis' experiments showed that supplemental vitamin C inhibited the formation of plaques in rabbits. These early results, demonstrating that vitamin C protects rabbits from atherosclerosis, have been confirmed and are not controversial.[39] The fact that vitamin C can inhibit plaque formation in rabbits is accepted,[40] although some experiments did not confirm the effect.[41] Other antioxidants, such as dietary vitamin E and selenium, also slow the development of atherosclerosis in rabbits.[42] The animal experiments support the idea that antioxidants, especially vitamin C, protect against heart disease and stroke.

If atherosclerosis is a form of scurvy, animals that lose the ability to synthesize vitamin C would develop plaques. A particular strain of laboratory mouse cannot produce vitamin C and possesses the same genetic defect as humans: both have a mutated gene for an enzyme called gulonolactone oxidase, needed to synthesize the vitamin. In the mouse, this deficiency can result in damage to the aorta,[43] the major blood vessel that carries blood away from the heart. The injury is not identical to human plaque, but our human ancestors lost the gene about 40 million years ago, whereas the experimental mouse lost it only recently. Unlike the mouse, people have had time to evolve protective mechanisms.

Another strain of mouse has very high cholesterol levels. Like some humans, this mouse does not have the ability to process cholesterol effectively and develops a form of atherosclerosis. Research has shown that feeding these mice vitamin C and other antioxidants can inhibit atherosclerosis.[44] Despite solid and increasing evidence that vitamin C can *protect* animals from atherosclerosis, this does not necessarily mean that vitamin C will *reverse* the disease.

REVERSING PLAQUES

It is easier to maintain health than to cure illness. Plaques, like other forms of chronic inflammation, may be difficult to eliminate once they become established. Scars are a permanent reminder of damage to the skin. Similarly, a healed atherosclerotic plaque may leave a damaged arterial wall, made solid with the deposition of calcium crystals.

Having shown that vitamin C might prevent atherosclerosis, Willis tried to reverse the illness in guinea pigs. He fed seventy-seven guinea pigs a diet low in vitamin C; then, after three to four weeks, he gave vitamin C to fifty of the animals. He inspected the remaining twenty-seven guinea pigs for signs of atherosclerosis. As controls, Willis fed twelve more guinea pigs the same diet, but with the addition of vitamin C.

Plaques did not develop in the controls that had received vitamin C throughout the experiment. More than half (sixteen) of the guinea pigs given the vitamin C-deficient diet without additional supplementation showed signs of atherosclerosis. Willis also found atherosclerosis in two-thirds (thirty-four) of the guinea pigs that had been given vitamin C after a month on the deficient diet. He claimed that when he fed vitamin C to his previously deprived guinea pigs, the small plaques healed quickly. He noted that immature plaques regressed following only two days of treatment. More advanced plaques, however, showed structural changes in the tissue that were more resistant to healing. His conclusion was that, while vitamin C prevents atherosclerosis in guinea pigs, it may only partially remove an existing plaque, leaving scar tissue behind.

Reversing Atherosclerosis in People?

Since Willis could partially reverse atherosclerosis in animals, he wondered if the same results were possible in people. In 1954, he began a study of the development of plaques in sixteen patients whose average age was 64 years old. Ten patients in the treatment group received 0.5 grams of vitamin C orally three times a day, while a control group of six patients did not receive supplemental vitamin C. Willis examined the patients' blood vessels using x-ray angiography,[45] taking repeated images of the same arteries, to monitor changes over time. He repeated the angiographies after periods of between two and six months. In the patients given supplemental vitamin C, Willis reported that plaques were becoming smaller and the patients' symptoms improved: six patients' plaques reduced in size and one patient's remained the same, although the remaining three showed continued plaque growth. The plaques also grew larger in two of the control patients; the other patients in the control group did not show any improvement in their disease or symptoms.

A criticism of Willis' research is that he gave too small a dose of vitamin C. A dose of 1.5 grams daily is not a large intake for a healthy person, let alone one with atherosclerosis. The intake now recommended to prevent a common cold, for example, is about 10 grams or more a day in divided doses. Despite this problem, Willis reported a direct beneficial effect in most of his patients.

Matthias Rath, a controversial former collaborator of Linus

Pauling, claims to have confirmed that some reversal of athero-sclerosis is possible. Rath used both vitamin C and an amino acid called lysine in his research. He measured arterial deposits in fifty-five subjects using an x-ray computed tomography (CT) body scanner. During the first six months of treatment, the therapy was reported to greatly reduce the growth of deposits.[46] Over the following six months, growth of arterial plaque in patients with early atherosclerosis ceased.

Taken alone, these results and those of Willis are not entirely convincing: either may have been a result of investigator bias. Nevertheless, they are consistent with the results of animal experiments and should therefore be taken seriously. Despite this, the response of corporate medicine has been to ignore the idea that heart disease and stroke may be a form of scurvy. Indeed, in addition to studying inadequate intakes, detractors have on occasion suggested vitamin C to be harmful. There is no evidence for harm and results that suggest large benefits have been either overlooked or disregarded.

VITAMIN C CLOGS ARTERIES?

Surprisingly, some members of the medical profession have advanced the view that rather than helping to prevent atherosclerosis, vitamin C promotes the disease. Proponents of the idea that vitamin C is harmful often cite the report that supplements might cause kidney stones; there is no evidence that this occurs with oral intakes. Here, we are specifically concerned with heart disease and will relate the odd case of a report that vitamin C supplements cause atherosclerosis.

A paper by Dr. James Dwyer and colleagues of the Los Angeles Atherosclerosis Study, presented at the 40th Annual Conference of the American Heart Association (March 2000), suggested that vitamin C clogs arteries.[47] The authors indicated that "regular use of vitamin C supplements may promote early atherosclerosis." This claim is not consistent with the main body of research on the vitamin. An earlier study, published by Dr. Stephen Kritchevsky, reported the opposite effect.[48] Kritchevsky measured the carotid artery wall in 6,318 women and 4,989 men, ranging from 45 to 64 years old. He found a significant *reduction* in thickness in people over 55 years of age who had consumed a gram or more of vitamin C each day. According to these results, higher intakes of vitamins C and E are linked to healthier artery walls.

Dwyer's results were incomplete and his assertion was premature, but the press splashed his claims across their pages, as is typical with reports that vitamins cause harm. These results were given a high profile in the mainstream media, which consistently neglects to cover genuine accounts of benefits provided by vitamins. Few people have heard that heart attack and stroke may be caused by too little vitamin C, for example. Dwyer's report was an oral presentation (not a journal paper) at a medical conference. Despite this, his alarming conclusion that vitamin C can be harmful was given international media coverage. According to Dwyer, people who had taken supplements of vitamin C for eighteen months had thicker carotid arteries—the measured increase in arterial wall thickness was reported to be 2.5 times that of the control subjects. Even if this were true, the results were incorrectly assumed to be bad news.

The description "increase in arterial thickness" is a relative value, of a kind which magnifies research results and makes them seem more important than is actually the case. Contrary to what many people assumed, the study did *not* report that the artery walls in those who took vitamin C were 2.5 times as thick as those of the controls. The value relates to a difference in the increase in wall thickness, over an eighteen-month period. The actual change in size could be so small as to be irrelevant. However, the presentation scared the media, along with readers who did not understand this distinction.

Dr. Paul Wand, a neurologist, investigated Dwyer's claim.[49] Earlier reports suggesting that vitamin C was protective against atherosclerosis used only the usual low doses. Wand found little information concerning doses greater than 2 grams of vitamin C per day, and his review showed that subjects taking over 500 milligrams per day were more likely to show a beneficial response than those taking less. Doses below 500 milligrams were not effective against cardiovascular disease.

REVIEW OF VITAMIN C AND CARDIOVASCULAR DISEASE		
	VITAMIN C DOSE < 500 MG	VITAMIN C DOSE > 500 MG
Beneficial response	1 study	30 studies
No response	3 studies	4 studies

Wand then conducted a pilot study with thirty subjects who had taken a minimum of 2 grams of vitamin C daily for at least four years, as well as other nutritional supplements. The subjects were older than those who participated in Dwyer's report, ranging in age from 45 to 81 years old, with an average age of 61 years. Wand measured the carotid artery thickness and the blood flow through the vessel with multiple scans, to see if plaque was present. This procedure allowed estimation of wall thickening, measurement of blood flow, and evidence of the degree of stenosis or blockage.

In his experiement, Wand observed that twenty-three out of thirty subjects who supplemented with high levels of vitamin C displayed no evidence of plaque formation, blockage, or wall thickening; they also had normal blood flow. There was some pathology in the remaining seven subjects—in five, the disease was insignificant, while the remaining two subjects had a degree of carotid blockage estimated at 30–40 percent. As these two subjects were of advanced age, this degree of blockage was considered normal. The seven cases with indications of carotid pathology had high levels of homocysteine, LDL cholesterol, or glucose. In other words, Wand's group of vitamin C supplement takers had remarkably healthy arteries. Rather than confirming harm, his results confirmed that vitamin C may prevent or even reverse atherosclerosis.

Wrong Without Explanation

Dr. Dwyer's claim was misleading and may have dissuaded people from supplementing with vitamin C. The study provided no evidence that vitamin C causes the carotid arteries to become blocked. Since blood flow was not measured, we do not have sufficient information to determine whether the change was detrimental or beneficial. More than two years after the conference presentation, the Dwyer study had still not been published, and when we asked, it was described as "under review."[50]

Dwyer's study was eventually published and claimed some antioxidants were *helpful* in preventing atherosclerosis. Moreover, it did not provide data to support the negative claims for vitamin C.[51] Indeed, the results contradicted the widely publicized claim that the vitamin is harmful! The paper presents results consistent with the idea that a high level of vitamin C (ascorbic acid) lowers both cholesterol and inflammation. The latter was measured using a high-sensitivity C-reactive protein test, hs-CRP. According to the report: "The water-soluble antioxidant, ascorbic acid [vitamin C], had a significant inverse association with total cholesterol (P = 0.006). The marker of chronic inflammation (hs-CRP) was significantly inversely related to plasma levels of ascorbic acid." This is the opposite of the claim for harm. The report also says: "Ascorbic acid [vitamin C] and tocopherols [vitamin E] were not significantly associated with IMT [intima media thickening] progression." This means there is no evidence that vitamin C caused arterial thickening, but rather that it lowers cholesterol and inflammation. So, it appears that the Los Angeles Atherosclerosis Study researchers made an incorrect claim to the media that vitamin C is harmful, though their final published results state the opposite.

Dwyer declined our request for additional evidence or explanation. The published results showed no significant relationship between vitamin C intake and thickening of the carotid artery. Moreover, they indicate potential benefit from large intakes. As far as we are aware, there was no explicit retraction of the earlier claims and the media neglected to inform the public that the over-hyped assertion—that vitamin C causes atherosclerosis—was simply wrong.

KEEPING ARTERIES HEALTHY

Taken alone, the animal experiments and limited clinical trials suggest that vitamin C may be beneficial in helping to prevent heart disease. Additional data indicates that vitamin C prevents arterial plaques in humans. In one study, the incidence of artery re-blockage following angioplasty was significantly reduced in fifty patients who were given 0.5 grams of vitamin C each day.[52] Angioplasty involves mechanical expansion using a small balloon to widen an obstructed blood vessel wall; the process damages the tissues and can promote rapid atherosclerosis.

In another study of rapid atherosclerosis, plaques were measured following heart transplants, using intravascular ultrasound. The researchers studied forty patients, who were given either 0.5 grams of vitamin C and 400 IU of vitamin E or a placebo, twice daily for a year.[53] The size of arterial plaques did not change in the vitamin-treated group but was found to increase by 8 percent in the placebo group. Additional research suggests that vitamins C and E slow arterial plaque growth in men.[54] A controlled study used two daily 250 milligram doses of vitamin C and 136 IU of vitamin E. Over three years, the combination was found to be effective, though these low doses of either vitamin alone were not. This suggests a synergistic benefit, as these antioxidants act together to fight free radicals. The beneficial effect continued over the following three years.[55] These results indicate that relatively low doses of supplements can slow progression of the disease.

In direct rebuttal of the claim in Dwyer's preliminary report, it appears that higher blood levels of vitamin C in men may be associated with *thinner* carotid artery walls.[56] Researchers measured the thickness of the arterial wall using ultrasound in 468 elderly men and women, aged 66–75 years, and found that the walls were less thick in men with higher plasma vitamin C concentration. Men with low vitamin E or beta-carotene levels were more likely to show carotid stenosis. This effect was not replicated in females, however. The authors of the study concluded that a high antioxidant vitamin status may help to prevent the initiation and progression of early atherosclerotic lesions in men.

The current evidence from epidemiological studies on vitamin C in the prevention of cardiovascular disease is debatable.[57] Some studies show a strong correlation between increased vitamin C intake and reduction of cardiovascular events, but others do not. Unfortunately, most studies of vitamin C and heart disease are indirect and have used inappropriately low doses. Typically, researchers measure blood levels of cholesterol or other risk factors, rather than measuring arterial plaque directly. Despite this limitation, there is solid supporting evidence that relatively low doses of vitamin C can inhibit arterial plaque formation,[58] though the research is not conclusive.[59] This epidemiologic confusion can be explained by the low doses studied and the inadequate frequency of dosing. The majority of studies employed a single daily dose of vitamin C, which is not frequent enough, given its half-life in the body of about thirty minutes.

Until the medical establishment conducts the appropriate high-dose clinical trials, people will need to decide for themselves, based on the evidence available. This suggests there is a real possibility that coronary heart disease and stroke are caused by lack of vitamin C, and there is little risk from taking supplements to maintain health.

SELECTIVE VISION

Early results on the effect of vitamin C on cardiovascular disease in animals have not been replicated adequately in humans. The preliminary animal studies have been repeated and the link between antioxidants and plaques in animals is well established: vitamin C prevents heart disease in animals. It may well be that high doses of vitamin C will have the same protective effect in humans.

We may wonder what Paterson and Willis would make of the apparent lack of interest in their research by the modern medical establishment. They presumably hoped and believed that their findings would be repeated, using solid clinical trials. Instead, over the following decades, billions of dollars have been spent on cholesterol research, despite the lack of evidence that cholesterol is a cause of atherosclerosis and heart disease. Meanwhile, the finding that feeding vitamin C to animals prevents development of atherosclerosis, even in the presence of high dietary cholesterol, has been ignored.

When Linus Pauling staked his reputation on the idea that vitamin C could prevent heart disease, he was impugned as a mere chemist who didn't realize that medicine was a practical discipline. Some critics claimed that his ideas might work in chemistry, but his approach could not benefit medicine. The detractors were apparently unaware that, far from being a novice in the field of medicine, Pauling had already made several contributions to the discipline, each of greater importance than the entire life's research of many of his faultfinders. Decades later, we are still waiting for medicine to investigate the idea that lack of vitamin C is responsible for the biggest killer in the industrialized nations.

It would be easy to test the action of vitamin C on atherosclerosis in humans. The blood vessel blockage could be measured in a small number of people with heart disease, before and after treatment with high-dose vitamin C or a placebo. Ultrasonic measurement of blood flow and wall thickness in the carotid artery would be a suitable direct physical measurement, easy to perform and noninvasive. While billions of dollars have been wasted on the medical fad of cholesterol, a possible cure may have been overlooked. Millions of people might be dying prematurely, for the lack of a few simple vitamin tablets.

THE PAULING THERAPY

Linus Pauling claimed that vitamin C could be used to cure heart disease.[60] He also devised a method of treatment that became known as the Pauling therapy:

• Vitamin C: 3–6 grams per day in divided doses

• Lysine: 3–6 grams per day in divided doses

• Proline: 0.5–2.0 grams per day in divided doses

The scientific basis of Pauling's therapy relies largely on the properties of vitamin C, though it also includes two amino acids, lysine and proline. These amino acids are normal components of proteins in the diet. Over the last decade, numerous people with heart disease have self-treated with vitamin C or the Pauling therapy.

Following from the work of Pauling's colorful collaborator, Matthias Rath, a particular form of "bad" cholesterol called lipoprotein(a) was suggested as an additional cause of heart disease. The Pauling and Rath model for heart disease claims that when there is not enough vitamin C, lipoprotein(a) is deposited in the arterial wall. The cholesterol thickens and strengthens the artery, repairing the damage caused by shortage of vitamin C. However, over time, the cholesterol ceases to be helpful and becomes harmful. As the illness continues, chronic inflammation sets in, the cholesterol becomes oxidized, and plaques form. The amino acid lysine acts against this process, by preventing the lipoproteins sticking to the artery wall.

Pauling suggested that, in times of deficiency, lipoprotein(a) cholesterol acts as a replacement for vitamin C.[61] During evolution, low levels of vitamin C in pre-humans might have caused scurvy and fragile blood vessels. Evolution might have favored individuals with an alternative method of strengthening their arteries, such as with lipoprotein(a) cholesterol. Although possible, this evolutionary argument is weak and cannot be tested scientifically.

It also implies that if sufficient vitamin C were present, the lipoprotein(a) would not be required to act as a surrogate.

Pauling and Rath claimed that the combination of vitamin C and lysine not only prevents atherosclerosis but also cures the disease by preventing lipoprotein(a) cholesterol from bonding to blood vessels.[62] There are a number of lysine binding sites in lipoprotein(a) that help it adhere within plaques and that may potentially have antioxidant properties. Lysine itself might compete with lipoproteins for access to binding sites in the artery wall. According to their patents,[63] a binding inhibitor such as lysine, used alone or with vitamin C, dissolves plaques. This explanation given for the Pauling therapy depends on another form of "bad" cholesterol[64] and diminishes the core idea of the action of vitamin C. The cholesterol association is unfortunate, but it led to Pauling's insight that lysine may help prevent cholesterol build-up in plaques.

The use of lysine to help dissolve arterial plaques is an interesting and important idea. However, this concept does not depend on a specific form of cholesterol, so the action of lysine should be considered separately from the involvement of lipoprotein(a). Both HDL and LDL cholesterol contain lysine residues.[65] Lysine could act on other forms of cholesterol to prevent plaque formation. If lysine prevents attachment, this would lessen the time it takes a lipoprotein particle to pass into and back out of the plaque. The decrease in transit time would lessen the chance of the lipoprotein being oxidized in the inflamed plaque. Even if it did become oxidized, it might leave the area quickly, without contributing to local inflammation. These mechanisms could combine to prevent plaque formation and help heal existing damage.

Regardless of this, the key idea remains that shortage of vitamin C may explain the prevalence of cardiovascular disease and most strokes.

IMPORTANT POINTS

- Unlike most animals, humans are singularly short of vitamin C.

- Most animals make their own vitamin C in large amounts and do not get heart disease.

- Atherosclerosis may be a result of chronic vitamin C deficiency.

- Large intakes of vitamin C could prevent or even reverse heart disease.

CHAPTER 11

VITAMIN E

"Unfortunately, everything the experts tell us about diet is aimed at the whole population, and we are not all the same."
—*THE SCIENTIST* MAGAZINE (SEPTEMBER 22, 2003)

Vitamin E is one of the most familiar antioxidants in the diet. Natural vitamin E is found in foods and, as described earlier, it consists of substances from two families of chemicals: tocopherols and tocotrienols. Unfortunately, the misconception that vitamin E is a single substance causes great confusion among scientists, medical professionals, and the public. It also leads to some inconsistent research findings. Suppose that on a Monday, research papers and the press report that "vitamin E" fails to prevent heart disease. The following day, they may cite research demonstrating that "vitamin E" does indeed prevent heart disease. By Wednesday, other researchers could present data that "vitamin E" has no effect on heart disease. Then, on Thursday, we might hear that "vitamin E" causes heart disease. By the end of the week, we could be reading that "vitamin E" is a powerful new treatment and can reverse atherosclerosis. Despite being contradictory, these reports could all be scientifically correct, as the results could relate to different forms of vitamin E.

Studies on "vitamin E" are scientifically weak, because the substance being studied could be any of a number of different chemicals, or even a mixture of different ones. As mentioned, synthetic vitamin E (dl-alpha-tocopherol) is a mixture of the d- and l-forms, together with numerous related molecules. Moreover, other chemicals, such as the supplement alpha-lipoic acid, also have vitamin E activity and can act as antioxidants in the body. So to reiterate, the name *vitamin E* refers to an action in the body, rather than to a particular substance. Vitamin E might be thought of as any of a number of antioxidants that prevent specified deficiency symptoms—although acute vitamin E deficiency is rare in humans. The various forms of vitamin E prevent the oxidation of fats in the body.[1]

Government nutritional recommendations are often arbitrary, rather than being based on science, which is strange considering the resources available to these organizations.[2] The U.S. Institute of Medicine and other organizations that have established recommended daily intakes appear to think that all forms of vitamin E are equal. They have based their standardization on a single molecule: alpha-tocopherol. However, all forms of vitamin E are not functionally identical. Both major families of vitamin E—tocopherols and tocotrienols—have their own specific properties,[2] which include acting as signaling molecules, shielding the body from cancer, and protecting against brain damage.[3]

VITAMIN E AND HEART DISEASE

Surveying the bulk of research on vitamin E brings to mind a quote by the physicist Wolfgang Pauli, who was known for his scathing remarks directed at his colleagues. Pauli once said of a theory: "It's not even wrong." This criticism might sound mild to a non-scientist, but we should remember that science depends fundamentally on refutation. Showing that an idea is wrong adds to the store of scientific knowledge, whereas an idea that is "not even wrong" cannot increase understanding at all. Many studies of "vitamin E" fall into the "not even wrong" category; they are not scientific.

For many years, health specialists have promoted the benefits of vitamin E for heart disease and atherosclerosis. Dr. Evan Shute and his brother, Dr. Wilfred Shute, became interested in the vitamin in 1936, when they explored its use as a treatment for heart disease and other problems. In those early days, the poor availability and quality of vitamin E preparations hindered their studies. Nonetheless, they obtained positive results, backing up their claims with clinical observations on thousands of patients over several decades, together with additional experimental results.[5]

Predictably, the medical establishment attacked both the Shutes and their results. In 1964, Herbert Bailey published a book called *Vitamin E: Your Key to a Healthy Heart*, in which he described how the medical establishment criticized the Shutes and suppressed their findings. Bailey wrote his book after suffering a heart attack, which he self-treated with vitamin E, following the Shutes' advice. Over the decades since the Shutes' original work, there have been many additional studies on the effects of relatively low doses of vitamin E on heart disease. While the results have not all been positive, the evidence suggests a protective effect—especially when vitamin E is used together with vitamin C.

The results of the Shutes' work have been partially confirmed, though the treatment is now thought to be less effective than originally suggested. The Cambridge Heart Antioxidant Study (CHAOS)[6] was an intervention-based clinical trial in which 2,002 heart patients were divided randomly into three groups and given either 400 IU or 800 IU of vitamin E (alpha-tocopherol) or a placebo, daily for 200 days. Both vitamin E groups showed a 77 percent decrease in incidence of non-fatal heart attack (14 out of 1,035 vitamin E subjects versus 41 out of 967 subjects who were not given a supplement), but there was no significant difference in the number of deaths. Another research group examined vitamin E and vitamin C supplementation in 11,178 elderly people, aged 67–105 years, from 1984 to 1993.[7] Supplementing with both vitamins, E and C, was associated with a lower risk of death from all causes and fewer deaths from coronary heart disease.

The well-known Harvard Medical School studies indicated that supplementation with more than 100 IU of vitamin E for more than two years decreased heart disease by 40 percent.[8] Subjects were 87,245 female nurses, 34–59 years old, in whom 552 cases of major coronary disease were noted over an eight-year period; and 39,910 male health professionals, 40–75 years old, in whom 667 cases of coronary disease were observed over a four-year period. The subjects had no previous history of heart disease. The male study also showed a positive effect for vitamin C, but this was not significant at the doses investigated.

The central importance of vitamin E is illustrated by the work of Fred Gey, who indicated that the most important risk factor for heart disease was a deficiency of vitamin E.[9] In each of the twelve countries he studied, vitamin E deficiency appeared to be of greater significance than a combination of smoking, blood pressure, and blood cholesterol.

DEFENDING THE PROFITS

Why have studies of benefits of vitamin E in heart disease been ignored by the medical and political establishments? Surely, it would be worthwhile to investigate an inexpensive treatment that might save many lives. Unfortunately, vitamin E and other supplements compete with the products of corporate medicine. People who choose supplements to prevent or treat heart disease might lower the sales of statins and other drugs. For this reason, claims that vitamins or other supplements are harmful abound in the media. Driving this negative hype is a series of clinical studies, often funded by corporate medicine. When these claims are given media focus—which is easily achieved, given the vast publicity budgets of the pharmaceutical industry—they create fear and mistrust of alternative medicine.

There have been claims that high intakes of vitamin E might cause a slight increase in mortality. A recent example is a review paper in the gold standard Cochrane Reviews, which claimed that antioxidant supplements have no beneficial effect.[10] Beta-carotene and vitamins A and E were reported to *increase* mortality. Doctors seized the opportunity to tell people not to take vitamins and supplements, particularly antioxidants.[11] Once again the claim that taking vitamin supplements could be deadly was picked up by the international media, flying around the world in no time at all.

Together with a number of international experts, we examined the report. The statistics were flawed[12] and the biology was unsound. The review selected its data in a biased way and was obviously misleading.[13] These criticisms have now been included by Cochrane in an update to the review. However, the authors and media have not retracted their alarmist claims. People might expect the media to exercise due diligence before being taken in by the vested interests of corporate medicine.

Eventually, such errors are corrected in the independent medical literature. In this case, two German scientists, Joachim Gerss and Wolfgang Köpcke, described the suggestion of harm in the review's title as "questionable" and "inconsistent." In the polite terms of scientific discourse, this amounts to a total rejection.[14] They explained that the result "can be explained by a higher proportion of male patients that were included in these trials compared to other trials" and that "none of these results can be regarded to supply evidence in a statistical sense." This claim that antioxidant vitamin supplements are harmful, like so many other transient media sensations, is nonsense.

MISTAKES OR MISINFORMATION?

The name tocopherol derives from the Greek, meaning "to bring forth offspring." Katharine Bishop and Herbert Evans discovered the vitamin E factor in 1922, when they found that rats raised purely on a diet of milk were unable to reproduce; their pups died in the womb. Provision of wheat germ and lettuce remedied the deficiency in the milk diet and, in the following years, the different vitamin E substances were identified.

The first question to ask with a vitamin E study is which form of the vitamin is being discussed. When this is done, the misleading claims from the media and corporate medicine appear obviously oversimplified. The tocopherols exist in a number of forms, called alpha-, beta-, gamma-, and delta-tocopherol. Each form of tocopherol has its own biological properties.[15] For example, mixed tocopherols can be stronger at protecting lipids from oxidation than alpha-tocopherol alone.[16] Alpha-tocopherol has some specific functions, such as signaling in arterial muscle cells.[17] Importantly, consumption of alpha-tocopherol can deplete blood levels of gamma-tocopherol.[18] The somewhat neglected gamma-tocopherol may be important, both for nutrition and for preventing atherosclerosis. Gamma-tocopherol possesses anti-inflammatory properties and high plasma concentrations may protect against cardiovascular disease[19] and prostate cancer.[20] Gamma-tocopherol is the most abundant form in the diet.

Synthetic vitamin E differs markedly from the natural forms. Many supplement takers have long ago rejected these synthetic vitamins. The natural forms are called d-alpha-, d-beta-, d-gamma-, and d-delta-tocopherol. It is commonly believed that synthetic vitamin E, dl-alpha-tocopherol, consists of a mixture of equal parts of the natural d- form and the biologically less active l- form. If this were the case, then some suggest it would be half as effective as d-alpha-tocopherol. However, synthetic alpha-tocopherol can exist in eight different forms, and only one of these unnatural forms—comprising 12.5 percent of the total mixture—is d-alpha-tocopherol; the other seven artificial forms have different molecular configurations and biological activities. When given to rats, the activities of these imitations range from 21 percent to 90 percent of d-alpha-tocopherol's activity.[21] In humans[22] and pigs,[23] the potency of synthetic alpha-tocopherol is lower than it is in rats. Notably, natural vitamin E produces higher blood levels.

Ideally, standard vitamin E supplements should be in the form of natural mixed tocopherols. The idea that synthetic substances can replace natural supplements, as claimed by the U.S. Institute of Medicine and other government regulatory bodies, is incorrect and potentially damaging to health.

THE OVERLOOKED VITAMIN

Another common form of "vitamin E" is particularly interesting for preventing and treating heart disease. Tocotrienols, found in rice and palm oils, are similar in structure to tocopherols but have a shorter side-chain that contains double bonds; this gives them different properties. As with tocopherols, there are several forms of tocotrienols: alpha-, beta-, gamma-, and delta-tocotrienol.[24] Like the tocopherols, the tocotrienols exist as optical isomers, in both d- and l- forms.

A general rule in biology is that each molecule has specific effects and actions. As with the tocopherols, the individual tocotrienols have particular biological activities. In rats, gamma-tocotrienol may lower blood pressure, prevent oxidation of fat in both blood and blood vessels, and improve the total antioxidant status.[25] In view of the distinctive properties of the tocotrienols, use of vitamin E supplements containing only alpha-tocopherol, whether for supplementation or for research, is even more questionable.[26] Thus, corporate medicine's claims for vitamin E, often based on synthetic alpha-tocopherol alone, are misleading in the extreme.

The biology of the different types of vitamin E varies greatly. Within cell membranes, tocotrienols spread out and disperse, whereas tocopherol molecules tend to clump together.[27] Some researchers have claimed that tocopherols are more powerful antioxidants; however, within body tissues, tocotrienols are more mobile than tocopherols and may be more biologically effective.[28] Additionally, tocotrienols may enter into tissues where tocopherols are largely absent. Furthermore, the tissue concentration, means of transport, and functions of tocopherols and tocotrienols in the body are different.[29] Tocotrienols are more effective at preventing brain damage[30] and brain cell death than their tocopherol cousins.[31] Perhaps most important to our discussion, however, is that tocotrienols may also be far more effective at preventing and treating cardiovascular disease.[32]

Tocotrienols are a superior type of vitamin E for preventing heart disease and may protect against atherosclerosis better than the more common forms of vitamin E. They inhibit white cell adhesion on the inner wall of arteries, caused by inflammation.[33] The greater effect of the tocotrienols arises because they accumulate in the endothelial cells lining the arterial walls, to levels tenfold greater than the tocopherols.[34] Notably, tocotrienols inhibit the formation of new blood vessel growth,[35] a characteristic of dangerous human plaques.

The less familiar form of vitamin E lowers the classic risk factors for heart disease and stroke. Tocotrienols appear to lower total blood cholesterol and low-density lipoprotein (LDL) cholesterol levels, and are also effective in preventing the oxidation of LDL cholesterol.[36,37] For those people who are interested in using statins, tocotrienols enhance the cholesterol-lowering effect of these medications.[38] However, alpha-tocopherol inhibits this action.[39]

While there are good theoretical and experimental reasons for using tocotrienols, we need results from patient studies in order to determine their utility in preventing and treating heart disease. These research results would be particularly convincing if they showed that existing disease could be reversed.

DISEASE REVERSAL

There is mounting evidence highlighting the benefits of antioxidants in protecting against cardiovascular disease. In 1992, scientists at the Atherosclerosis Laboratory at the University of Mississippi demonstrated the use of antioxidant supplements to prevent and reverse atherosclerosis in monkeys.[40] Soon afterwards, studies with humans indicated that antioxidants could slow the progression of atherosclerosis.[41] Researchers studied 100 patients who had undergone coronary angioplasty, a procedure to stretch atherosclerotic blood vessels in the heart.[42] As we have described, such interventions damage the arterial wall and can create rapid local atherosclerosis. The patients were given either a large dose of vitamin E or a placebo daily. Four months later, restenosis, which is re-narrowing of the arteries because of plaque buildup, was found in about half the placebo subjects but only one-third of those supplementing with vitamin E.

Vitamin E can reverse heart disease. In mice and rabbits fed unnaturally large amounts of cholesterol, tocotrienols protect the arteries from thickening and damage,[43] although the effect may take weeks to develop fully.[44] Tocotrienols have been shown to reduce the arterial blockage caused by plaque and arteriosclerosis. In a three-year, double-blind clinical study, cardiologist Marvin Bierenbaum showed that tocotrienols can lead to regression of atherosclerosis.[45] Bierenbaum's research group observed that tocopherols and tocotrienols greatly reduced activity in the platelets and could prevent clots from forming. Platelets are small, disc-shaped particles in the blood that accumulate in large numbers at the site of an injured blood vessel.

Since tocotrienols had been shown to reduce the effects of dietary cholesterol in rats, Bierenbaum decided to try them in humans. In 1995, his research group measured the effects of both gamma-tocotrienol and alpha-tocopherol on carotid atherosclerosis. The study estimated the degree of carotid artery blockage over eighteen months, in fifty patients with cerebrovascular disease. Ultrasound scans of the artery were done at six months and twelve months, and continued yearly.

The results of Bierenbaum's study indicated that tocotrienols reduce blood vessel blockage. Initially, tocotrienols reversed the disease in a little over a quarter of the patients. Ultrasound measurements revealed improvement in seven of the twenty-five patients given gamma-tocotrienol and progression in two. None of the control group of twenty-five patients showed improvement. Ten untreated patients showed increased disease and blockage.

Blood platelet oxidation decreased in the treatment group after twelve months, but the placebo group showed an increase, although it was not significant. Blood levels of LDL ("bad") cholesterol, HDL ("good") cholesterol, and triglycerides remained unchanged. This implies that plaques can be reversed independently of the level of blood cholesterol, further demolishing the outdated mainstream idea that high cholesterol causes heart disease. The effect of the tocotrienols increased with time and ultimately provided benefits in almost all patients. In a later report, 92 percent of the patients in the tocotrienol group were reported as stabilized or improved; in the control group, 48 percent of the patients deteriorated and none of the patients improved.

Bierenbaum suggested that oxidized cholesterol exists in both stable and mobile pools within an arterial plaque. Tocotrienols prevent oxidation of cholesterol in the loose pool and help move it out of the artery wall, before it can become attached to the plaque. This mechanism clarifies the dramatic effects for patients who were given tocotrienols, which suggested a cure after only six months of treatment. The reversal of plaques with tocotrienols depends on their action as local antioxidants, and it is consistent with the antioxidant effect described for vitamin C. Indeed, the hypothesis that tocotrienols prevent cholesterol molecules sticking in plaque is similar to that for the action of vitamin C and lysine, proposed by Linus Pauling (see Chapter 10).

Animal studies have confirmed the potential benefits of tocotrienols on heart disease. Certain mice with a genetic defect in lipid processing develop atherosclerosis, when fed a high-cholesterol diet. A study of these mice found that tocotrienols inhibited plaque formation.[46] Mice that were not given supplements developed large plaques at the level of their aortic valves. In contrast, mice given a tocotrienol supplement had plaques that were 92–98 percent smaller. In other words, the control mice had large plaques and the treated mice had almost insignificant plaques. This difference in the size of the plaques occurred despite the finding that treated mice had similar blood fat levels to the controls. A second research group, working on a similar strain of mice, confirmed and extended these results.[47]

In a further study, eighteen rabbits were fed an unnatural, cholesterol-rich diet for ten weeks. The results suggested that tocotrienols could have beneficial effects on blood lipids and reduce oxidation in arteries.[48] A second rabbit study, carried out over a twelve-week period, indicated that tocotrienols provided greater protection against plaque formation than the more common tocopherol form of vitamin E.[49]

If corporate medicine announced results of this magnitude from a new drug, there would be a media frenzy. The statin "wonder" drugs simply do not compare. There is strong evidence that cardiovascular disease is reversible and people do not need to die prematurely. Moreover, such results might be expected from basic biology. People get heart disease because of a slight imbalance in their physiology; this cause has been sufficiently obscure for corporate medicine to have failed to find it. The idea that prevention and treatment could result from a simple change in diet may be an affront to some, but it is what the evidence suggests.

FAST-MOVING ANTIOXIDANTS

Two independent lines of research, based on two different vitamins, indicate that antioxidants can reverse atherosclerosis. Why do vitamin C and the tocotrienols seem to work, when other antioxidants, such as the tocopherol forms of vitamin E, do not? A likely explanation is that the beneficial supplements are mobile molecules that can penetrate the plaque in sufficient quantities to have the desired effect. Having acted as an antioxidant, the molecule can leave the tissue and be replaced. Conversely, while supplements of many other antioxidants accumulate in the blood, they do not appear to enter plaques at high levels, are less mobile and therefore ineffective.[50]

At first glance, tocotrienols appear to be more effective than vitamin C in treating atherosclerosis. However, this may result from a lack of studies using high-dose vitamin C. Bierenbaum's clinical study with tocotrienols covered a longer period than the six-month studies on vitamin C and plaques conducted by Willis and Rath (see Chapter 10). Additionally, vitamin E is fat-soluble and stays in the body for a longer period than vitamin C. The possibility remains that large dynamic flow intakes of vitamin C, taken over a longer duration, could be more effective than tocotrienols. However, since both high dose vitamin C and tocotrienols may operate by the same antioxidant mechanism, there exists the exciting prospect that they could be synergistic.

Given these findings, why did the world's media not immediately announce the curative potential of tocotrienols? Author and nutritional scientist, Richard Passwater, interviewed Bierenbaum and asked him why he did not make more of his potentially important results. His reply intimated that this was the age of the megastudy and the meta-analysis of results from several large studies. Because Bierenbaum's study included only fifty patients, he suggested that it was considered less "solid" evidence than a megastudy. If this really is the case, then medical science has lost its way. Validation in science comes from replication. If you are looking for a reliable cure for heart disease, you will find it with a small study like Bierenbaum's, followed by replication. Some people speculate that pharmaceutical companies are reluctant to conduct follow-up studies, because they would lose billions of dollars in drug sales if these findings were confirmed.

Vitamin C and tocotrienols can reverse coronary heart disease. An important question is whether high-dose vitamin C and tocotrienols, supplied together, would work synergistically in an antioxidant network. If so, a combination of high-dose vitamin C and tocotrienols would be appropriate for removing arterial plaques. People cannot assume that corporate medicine will provide unbiased advice. Decide for yourself and do your own cost-benefit analysis. On the available evidence, the combination of high-dose vitamin C and tocotrienols could be curative and has no known harmful effects.

IMPORTANT POINTS

- Antioxidants that can move easily through tissues are more effective.

- Some forms of vitamin E are unlikely to be effective antioxidants, unless intake is high.

- Most studies of vitamin E have used inadequate doses or have used the wrong form.

- The tocotrienol form of vitamin E appears to be effective in reversing arterial plaques.

- Vitamin C and tocotrienols could provide an effective treatment—or even a cure—for atherosclerosis.

CHAPTER 12

NO MORE FEAR

"Everyone now has a choice, a clear choice."
—LOUIS J. IGNARRO

Governments and medical authorities warn repeatedly about the risk factors associated with cardiovascular disease and, as a result, many people are in a state of anxiety when considering their options. That pain in your chest may be a stomach ache, but what if it is the heart attack you have been dreading? You may worry that overexertion or a stressful job could lead to heart problems. This fear is heightened when a friend your age (or even a little younger) needs a triple bypass operation, or you read a newspaper article about a young athlete who dropped dead from a heart attack.

All this worry is a waste of effort and energy! You may need only a few easy preventive measures to keep your cardiovascular system healthy as you age. Atherosclerosis is not inevitable or compulsory: it can be avoided. By now, you should understand that risk factors do not cause the disease. Rather, heart disease is a symptom of modern living—largely attributable to poor nutrition and smoking tobacco.

In this chapter, we explain how supplementing your diet can reduce your risk of atherosclerosis and associated events, such as stroke and heart attack. In high enough doses, specific nutrients may even reverse the disease. By supplementing their diet, people with atherosclerosis and related cardiovascular disease might restore themselves to something like normal health.

To begin, the protocols for *prevention* and *treatment* of heart disease are not the same. In the first case, the person is presumably healthy and merely wishes to avoid heart disease or stroke in the future. In the second, the person has already experienced some degree of atherosclerosis and wants to reverse the disease process. It should not come as any surprise that treatment of an existing disease requires a more intensive approach than prevention.

STANDARD PREVENTION OF HEART DISEASE

For a healthy person, prevention of heart disease requires a minimum of about 3 grams of vitamin C, spread throughout the day. This would be equivalent to 1 gram every eight hours. Lower intakes than this minimum dynamic flow level are unlikely to be effective. Some people will have higher requirements because they are at greater susceptibility. This minimal intake is enough to ensure that deficiency does not occur (unless a person is stressed or sick); it can be achieved easily by taking 1 gram of vitamin C with every meal.

It is not worth paying excessive prices for special forms of vitamin C—simple, inexpensive ascorbic acid is adequate. However, if you find the acid form of vitamin C causes stomach irritation, you could try sodium ascorbate or magnesium ascorbate. Magnesium ascorbate is a good option, as many people are also deficient this mineral.

In addition to vitamin C, a daily multivitamin tablet containing the range of B vitamins, and a variety of dietary antioxidants, such as natural vitamin E and coenzyme Q_{10}, are helpful in preventing heart disease.

PREVENTION FOR THOSE AT HIGHER RISK

People who are currently healthy but who could be at risk of heart disease (perhaps because it is common in their family) might consider at least doubling the intake of vitamin C, to 6–10 grams a day. These dynamic flow intakes, and even larger levels, are considered safe.

Some people have difficulty taking high doses of standard vitamin C because of their bowel tolerance limit. Healthy people get loose stools if they consume too high a dose. Splitting the dose into several smaller doses, taken at intervals (say, every four hours), may overcome the problem. Another approach is to take half the dose as standard tablets and half as liposomal vitamin C. This combination can increase blood levels of vitamin C, because the two forms are absorbed independently.

People at particularly high risk of heart disease may consider adding daily doses of mixed natural tocotrienols (250+ milligrams), along with extra tocopherols (800+ IU), and R-alpha-lipoic acid (100–200 milligrams, three times a day). Note that the naturally occurring R-form of alpha-lipoic acid (R-ALA) is more physiologically available than synthetic S- or mixed R/S- forms. Alpha-lipoic acid can degrade easily, so it should be stored in a cool, dry place. Importantly, the sodium (Na-RALA) and potassium salts (K-RALA) are more stable and are more effective as supplements.

The inclusion of lysine and proline, as suggested by Linus Pauling, may be justified, as they have low toxicity and could be beneficial. The Antioxidant Network Therapy regime for prevention, shown in the table on page 190, is similar to the Pauling Therapy, but includes additional antioxidant support, in the form of natural vitamin E, tocotrienols, and alpha-lipoic acid.

ANTIOXIDANT NETWORK THERAPY

Based on current evidence, we provide an extension to Pauling's original approach, which we have called Antioxidant Network Therapy. As mentioned above, it is vital to be specific about the differences between prevention and treatment. Pauling's idea was

PAULING THERAPY COMPARED WITH ANTIOXIDANT NETWORK THERAPY		
	PAULING THERAPY	ANTIOXIDANT NETWORK THERAPY
Vitamin C	3–6 grams	At or near bowel tolerance: 6+ grams
Liposomal vitamin C	N/A	Equal to or above standard vitamin C intake
Lysine	3–6 grams	3–6 grams
Proline	0.5–2.0 grams	0.5–2.0 grams
Tocotrienols	—	300+ mg
Tocopherols	—	800+ IU
R-alpha-lipoic acid	—	300–600 mg

that taking vitamin C and the amino acid lysine would prevent or cure heart disease. His approach also included niacin (vitamin B$_3$) and an anti-clotting agent (tranexamic acid). His central idea, however, was that atherosclerosis is caused by too little vitamin C in the diet.

A weakness of the Pauling/Rath theory of heart disease is its reliance on the form of cholesterol called lipoprotein(a), which was considered to build up inside arterial walls, strengthening the vessel and acting as an antioxidant. This is a plausible explanation for the buildup observed in arterial plaque, but limiting the idea to a single form of cholesterol is restrictive. This inclusion of cholesterol may have arisen from the earlier work of Matthias Rath, accommodated into the approach by Pauling. It also acknowledges the current obsession with cholesterol and heart disease; Pauling may have thought it might make the idea more palatable to mainstream medicine. It did not. The cholesterol aspect of the model detracts from the primary message: atherosclerosis is caused by a shortage of antioxidants, particularly vitamin C.

TREATMENT FOR EXISTING ATHEROSCLEROSIS

Drastic action is needed to eliminate existing atherosclerotic plaques. Thus, in most cases, Linus Pauling's suggested doses of vitamin C are too small for clinical benefit: *dynamic flow levels* are needed. Robert Cathcart's bowel tolerance method might be more suitable. The late Dr. Cathcart worked with us to originate the dynamic flow concept. He had previously described how a person's intake of vitamin C was limited by its laxative effect. Rather than seeing this as an unwanted side effect, Cathcart noticed that bowel tolerance increases when a person is sick. As he pointed out, the changing bowel tolerance level provides an indicator of how much vitamin C a person needs to be healthy. In general, the sicker people are, the more vitamin C they can absorb.

Producing a dynamic flow level of vitamin C involves gradually increasing the amount taken, until the intake causes loose stools, then just backing off slightly. The doses should be spread throughout the day (every 4–6 hours). If taken all at once, a large dose is more likely to have a powerful laxative effect. Spreading out the dose is both physiologically and financially more efficient, as it allows more of the vitamin to be absorbed. It is also important to maintain a flow of vitamin C through the body. Based on the bowel tolerance method, the resulting vitamin C dose will vary, both between people and for the same person at different times. However, this method is likely to result in a dose that is appropriate to the person's individual biochemical and physiological needs.

Liposomal vitamin C is becoming widely available and provides a way of increasing the benefits of oral intakes. Reversing atherosclerosis is difficult and liposomes may offer lifesaving benefits. However, liposomal vitamin C is a more expensive form of oral intake. To lower the cost and maximize the benefit, take the liposomes on top of dynamic flow levels of standard vitamin C. Reversing atherosclerosis is difficult and, in some cases, the liposomal form of the vitamin may be essential to maintain the high intake required.

Contraindications to high-dose supplementation of vitamin C will be described shortly (see the section on Dynamic Flow Vitamin C). Additional safety considerations apply with the other supplements, such as high dose R-alpha-lipoic acid. There may be further factors for an individual and, as with any treatment, this regime should only be considered with medical advice.

In cases of existing disease, at least six months of treatment with either Antioxidant Network Therapy or Pauling Therapy will be needed before plaque reduction is likely to become apparent. We would expect to see some plaque reduction within one year of starting antioxidant network treatment and would predict the full effect within two years.

IS ANTIOXIDANT THERAPY PROVEN?

The evidence we have considered in this book is not conclusive: it does not "prove" that vitamin C or other antioxidants, such as vitamin E as tocotrienols, will prevent or cure atherosclerosis. As we have explained, claims and demands for proof are not scientific. Real science does not involve proof. Ask anyone who makes such an irrational demand to read Karl Popper's book *The Logic of Scientific Discovery*. In the words of Karl Popper, "Whenever a theory appears to you as the only possible one, take this as a sign that you have neither understood the theory nor the problem which it was intended to solve." We do not offer proof, only rationality.

Linus Pauling suggested that his treatment could cure heart disease. The medical profession tends to avoid the word "cure" as too strong a claim. For example, treatment with insulin does not cure diabetes, but converts it to a long-term, degenerative condition. Some critics suggest that one reason for avoiding the word is that curing a continuing condition goes against the financial interests of pharmaceutical and related industries. An ongoing "treatment" for a chronic condition is more profitable than a one-off cure. However, there is another explanation: the conversion of medicine to genetic and social studies, such as epidemiology, means that cures have been replaced by the now-ubiquitous "risk factors." Finding cures is apparently just too great a challenge for corporate medicine.

Despite this, antioxidant therapy may indeed be curative, as Pauling and others have suggested. In the past, scurvy was a widespread and fatal disease, which was cured by vitamin C. The definition of a vitamin is that its absence from the diet will cause a disease. So, for example, absence of niacin (vitamin B_3) causes pellagra, and a diet with sufficient niacin can cure it. Vitamins cure their associated deficiency diseases. Atherosclerosis and heart disease may be signs of chronic scurvy. If this is the case, then providing sufficient vitamin C would cure the disease.

We do not know for certain that atherosclerosis is a form of long-term scurvy and neither does the medical profession. More importantly, they appear to have little interest in finding out. For over half a century, reputable scientists and physicians have proposed theories and provided suggestive evidence concerning the cause and possible cures for the biggest killers in the Western world. It is almost unbelievable that medical science has utterly failed to test these and people have continued to die from a disease that could, like the acute scurvy of the olden days, turn out to be preventable.

TOP TEN SUPPLEMENTS

We prefer low-cost approaches to maintaining health, as we feel that too many people in the field of corporate medicine build extravagant lifestyles at the expense of the sick. Eating a healthy diet is one of the most cost-effective ways to avoid becoming a medical statistic. For example, lowering your intake of fructose has zero cost: simply cut out those food products with added sugar (fructose or sucrose) and high-fructose corn syrup. If you have a sweet tooth, you can use glucose or stevia as safer alternatives to artificial sweeteners. In excluding fructose and sucrose,

STOPPING INFLAMMATION NATURALLY

Anti-inflammatory drugs have largely been a failure in cardiovascular disease. This dismal result is not because the drugs fail to inhibit inflammation, but because they possess unfortunate side effects. To prevent cardiovascular disease, a drug needs to be taken every day, for decades. A first approximation is that the side effects are proportional to the total dose consumed. Over time, massive doses of a drug such as aspirin can irritate your stomach and erode your joints.

The classic case of an anti-inflammatory drug gone wrong is Vioxx (rofecoxib). This drug was given to over 80 million people, but was rapidly withdrawn from the market when long-term use was found to *increase* heart attacks and strokes. Vioxx and its cousin, Celebrex, are selective nonsteroidal, anti-inflammatory drugs (NSAIDs), which may be thought of as improved forms of aspirin. Their mechanism of action is essentially a copy of some herbal remedies, in particular, turmeric (curcumin). The new drugs promised to give relief from inflammation, without aspirin's side effects. Unlike turmeric, however, Vioxx delivered large financial rewards (billions of dollars a year) for the drug company that developed it. Vioxx had just one problem—it killed many thousands of the patients who were prescribed it.

People can use natural supplements to prevent chronic inflammation. Turmeric is safe and has been used as a spice for hundreds of years—it is what gives curry its yellow color. Turmeric has the same mechanism of action as the drugs that were presumably designed to be profitable copies. So it may seem puzzling why so many people risk taking some rather dangerous drugs, rather than a tasty spice that has an equivalent action and fewer side effects. However, the culture of modern medicine is to denigrate natural remedies, in order to gain massive profits. Your doctor is unlikely to suggest using turmeric instead of the latest Vioxx-type drug. Indeed, a person is more likely to be told not to take supplements of curcumin, turmeric's main active ingredient. After all, curcumin might be dangerous, say the doctors, without a hint of irony.

Three anti-inflammatory herbs may be considered as a starting point to prevent the inflammation associated with atherosclerosis: curcumin, ginger, and *Boswellia.* Most people are familiar with turmeric (curcumin) and ginger, and these are generally regarded as safe. Curcumin is particularly effective as an antioxidant and anti-inflammatory, but it is not well absorbed when taken orally. However, BCM-95 or similar forms are available, which offer greatly improved absorption. *Boswellia* is the frankincense mentioned in the Bible; it is widely used in Ayurvedic medicine. Clearly, its use has a long history. Supplements of these and other herbs are available, as are the herbs themselves. Use the spices liberally and follow the recommendations of the manufacturer and your physician.

you will find yourself forced to eat a healthier diet and to avoid junk food.

Rather than start at the number one supplement, we have elected to begin with the issue of smoking. Smoking tobacco is a wholesale assault on the cells and tissues of the body. In particular, it irritates the arterial walls, generates inflammation, and promotes arterial disease. These things are bad enough, but smoking also prevents the action of life-saving nutrients.

Large intakes of antioxidants, such as vitamin C, can prevent or reverse atherosclerosis. However, it is difficult to get the antioxidants into the artery wall to where they can help. Smoking fills the bloodstream with oxidants and free radicals, putting a severe strain on the protective antioxidants. In smokers, most of the antioxidants in the diet will be consumed in quenching the smoking-induced free radicals, before they can even reach the artery walls to fight atherosclerosis.

This is not intended as nannying advice—people should be free to choose to smoke or not. However, the decision to smoke may negate much of the help provided by nutrient supplements and be financially expensive. It seems that the choice to smoke really does mean accepting the associated risks of heart disease, cancer, and other diseases. The decision not to smoke means that not only do you reap immediate health (and financial) benefits, but you can then lower your risk of atherosclerosis to negligible levels by taking supplements.

Here, we list ten important supplements for preventing atherosclerosis, heart attack, and stroke. The order reflects a combination of importance and cost.

#1   Dynamic Flow Vitamin C

Take dynamic flow levels of vitamin C. Levels vary from person to person but, in an average healthy individual, dynamic flow starts when the person takes about 3 grams of vitamin C each day. Thus, a person wishing to prevent heart disease might consume 1 gram (1,000 milligrams) of vitamin C with each meal. A few people find they need to build up to this level of intake. If you are one of these, you might start with 500 milligrams per day and gradually increase the frequency and dose until you are taking 1 gram three times daily.

Most people can safely consume large intakes of vitamin C; the main side effect with a high intake is its laxative action. If loose stools become a problem, then the dose can simply be lowered slightly. People with iron overload disease, kidney disease, or glucose-6-phosphatase deficiency (a rare condition) should consult their doctor before taking high doses. However, the real "side effect" of high intakes of vitamin C is greatly improved health.

Contrary to popular and medical opinion, five fruits or vegetables a day will not help greatly. This suggestion was aimed at getting people to take 200 milligrams of vitamin C each day. However, the advice was based on a misunderstanding that a person could not absorb more than 200 milligrams of vitamin C in a day. In fact, most healthy individuals can absorb up to 20,000 milligrams of vitamin C a day and some may need these high intakes to maintain health. The official guidelines (Recommended Dietary Allowance or RDA) for vitamin C need urgent revision: the quoted daily requirement is at least ten times too low. The minimum healthy intake is probably above 2,000 milligrams a day.

A 3 or 4 gram daily intake of vitamin C is adequate for most healthy people, who are not at high risk of heart disease. Those who have a particular risk may consider taking more. Higher intakes are appropriate for people with existing symptoms or those from families whose members have suffered heart disease, atherosclerosis, or stroke. Other people at risk may be those suffering from type 2 diabetes. Some people simply have a higher-than-average requirement for vitamin C—you can tell this by finding your bowel tolerance level: if it is high, your body is asking for more. Remember, your bowel tolerance will vary as your health does. An intake of 10–12 grams a day (say, 3 grams with each of four daily meals) is a minimum for people at risk.

In people with greater need, the intake required may be higher than can be achieved with standard vitamin C. Adding liposomal vitamin C to near bowel tolerance levels of the standard preparation will enable higher intakes and, consequently, higher blood levels to be achieved, without the usual bowel tolerance limitations.

If it is true that atherosclerosis is a result of chronic scurvy, then these intakes of vitamin C will prevent atherosclerosis, coronary heart disease, and occlusive stroke. It is possible that this vitamin C regimen could eliminate most cardiovascular disease.

#2   The Right Kinds of Vitamin E

From the 1930s, Dr. Wilfred Shute and Dr. Evan Shute, in Canada, reported the benefits of vitamin E in cardiovascular disease.[1] The benefits described by the Shutes with the d-alpha-tocopherol form of vitamin E were not fully supported by later studies. It is possible that the population that the Shutes studied was depleted in the vitamin. Whatever the reason, when studies are repeated, initial reports of a large benefit are often found to be smaller. In this case, later studies demonstrated a reduction in heart disease of 30–40 percent, with vitamin E intakes up to 800 IU per day. However, with appropriate levels of supplementation and with the more effective forms of vitamin E, the potential benefits may be as large as—or even greater than—the Shutes initially reported.

Choose your vitamin E carefully: the doses of most vitamin E supplements are too low for it to act as an antioxidant. Many are synthetic forms and are probably close to useless. The standard rule for vitamin E is to get mixed natural tocopherols (d-form); at least 1,600 IU a day is needed to provide a reasonable anti-oxidant effect. Our suggestion is lower because of the addition of tocotrienols.

Tocotrienols are important: experiments suggest that this less common form of vitamin E may reduce arterial plaque and reverse atherosclerosis. To prevent coronary disease, 250 milligrams daily of mixed tocotrienols is a reasonable intake. Healthy people at higher risk can take more, perhaps 250–500 milligrams daily. Those with existing arterial disease might consider taking 500–1,000 milligrams a day. The tablets can be taken with a fish oil capsule to aid absorption. If possible, avoid taking tocotrienols at the same time as standard vitamin E, as tocopherols can inhibit their absorption.

We have placed the tocotrienols at number two in our list, reflecting their importance. Indeed, for those wishing to reverse existing cardiovascular disease, the tocotrienols may be even more effective than high intakes of vitamin C. The appropriate trials have not been performed to say this with any certainty, however. To get the best of both worlds, people can take vitamin C and tocotrienols together and thus gain increased benefit from any possible synergies. This approach may even reverse chronic athero-sclerosis.

#3   B-100

The B-group vitamins can be taken together as a single high-dose "B-100" tablet. Taking a B-100 tablet will lower blood levels of homocysteine, which is considered a new "risk factor" for cardio-vascular disease. However, lowering homocysteine may not have any direct effect on preventing heart disease; as with other risk factors, it is only a *marker* that is in some way associated with the illness, not a direct cause of the disease. High blood levels of homocysteine indicate that a person is deficient in B vitamins. In particular, the person may have low levels of pyridoxine (vitamin B_6), folic acid (vitamin B_9), and cyanocobalamin (vitamin B_{12}). In this case, high homocysteine indicates that deficiencies of B vitamins are implicated in cardiovascular disease.

Deficiency of vitamin B_{12} is endemic. There is a good chance that the reader is deficient in this nutrient, even if they are taking a high-dose B-complex supplement (B-100). Vitamin B_{12} is most-ly found in animal products, so vegetarians and vegans can become deficient.[4] Also, because B_{12} is attached to animal proteins and is released by gastric enzymes and stomach acid, people who use long-term antacid medications may lower their absorption of this vitamin. Absorption is typically poor, though the human body pro-vides a protein called intrinsic factor to help its uptake. About one in fifty people over sixty years of age have some degree of perni-cious anemia, which reduces B_{12} absorption, as intrinsic factor is depleted.[5] Surveys indicate that at least one in twenty are vitamin B_{12}–deficient, with the prevalence increasing with age.[6] About one in five have marginal deficiency later in life.

Blood levels used to indicate Vitamin B_{12} deficiency may be far too low and such deficiency could be a cause of chronic disease. Vitamin B_{12} deficiency is linked to a number of major conditions, such as dementia,[2] as well as cardiovascular disease.[3] Taking extra vitamin B_{12} is safe and may help prevent coronary disease and other chronic conditions. While oral absorption is often limited, high doses can overcome the restriction. In particular, the use of sublingual tablets, held under the tongue or next to the gum, can help improve absorption.

People on a normal diet with no particular concern about coronary disease may be well served by a B-100 tablet. A low-cost B-100 tablet will ensure that sufficient B vitamins are present in the diet to avoid an unnecessary risk of heart disease. Try to find a sustained-release B-100 tablet, as most B vitamins are excreted relatively rapidly. Vegans, vegetarians, and those with a specific concern about heart disease can elect to take a weekly sublingual B_{12} tablet, say 1,000–5,000 µg (1–5 milligrams), in addition to their B-complex supplement. Those with existing atherosclerosis might take 1 milligram of B_{12} sublingually each day. Once again, these high intakes are not only considered safe but may have additional health benefits.

#4   Niacin

Vitamin B_3 (niacin) is required in larger amounts than the other B vitamins and needs to be considered separately. In large doses, it is a treatment for high cholesterol levels. Intakes of 1,000–2,000 milligrams, taken three or four times daily (a total of 4–6 grams per day), may be more effective than the overhyped statin drugs. Niacin is unique: it raises "good" HDL cholesterol and lowers "bad" LDL cholesterol.

Niacin helps maintain the arterial wall and prevents atherosclerosis. Some of the effects of niacin may be related to its side-effect of skin flushing. Although it may at first feel as though you are on fire, the short periods of dramatic skin flushing that are experienced with high dose niacin tend to fade with repeated use; some people even learn to enjoy them. If not, flushing can be minimized by taking niacin with a meal. Low-flush forms of vitamin B_3 are available, but these may not be as effective for maintaining cardiovascular health. It is also more cost-effective to use the cheaper niacin form of vitamin B_3, rather than the more expensive low-flush or no-flush forms.

The usual explanation for the use of statins and other expensive drugs, as opposed to niacin, relate to the reported side effects of niacin, such as rare cases of liver damage. However, Dr. Abram Hoffer, who had the most clinical experience in this area, reported that his patients, who were given niacin with high levels of antioxidants, did not have these problems.

As with all interventions, you should check with your doctor to see if you are at particular risk before taking high doses of niacin. Most people can tolerate large intakes with a high degree of safety. High intakes of niacin may be combined with high intakes of vitamin C and a B-100 tablet.

#5 Magnesium

Magnesium deficiency is commonplace: two in every three people in the United States do not even meet the government's suggested intake level. This mineral is often overlooked in favor of its close and more abundant relative, calcium. However, like calcium, magnesium is an essential element and is involved in hundreds of biochemical reactions in our bodies. Deficiency may contribute to atherosclerosis, heart disease and stroke. In addition, magnesium deficiency is associated with diabetes, high blood pressure, migraine, osteoporosis, and anxiety disorders. Low levels of magnesium can promote inflammation and increase LDL cholesterol levels.[10]

With conventional medicine's bias toward the cholesterol model, the connection between magnesium and heart disease has been mostly overlooked. Magnesium has multiple beneficial effects on the cardiovascular system and offers an effective and safe first-line treatment for heart problems, such as arrhythmias and ventricular tachycardia.[8] It provides a safe treatment for eclampsia (hypertension) and pre-eclampsia in pregnancy. Magnesium sulfate more than halves the risk of eclampsia and lowers the risk of maternal death.[9] In this role, it is more effective and safer than some commonly used drugs.

Epsom salts include magnesium sulfate. These well-known bath salts, renowned for their health-giving properties, get their name from the English town of Epsom, now part of greater London. The original salts were obtained by boiling the local mineral water. Magnesium sulfate is a common ingredient in modern bath salts. Because magnesium absorption from diet and supplements is limited, some claim that bathing in Epsom salts or other salts with a high magnesium content can help.[7] Bath salts are often promoted for muscular aches and pains, and for general relaxation. Similarly, Epsom salts may be used as a treatment for skin disorders, such as boils and abscesses, which like atherosclerosis are associated with inflammation.

Supplementation requires a little care: the common form, magnesium oxide, is poorly absorbed and may be considered as a laxative. Magnesium absorption from supplements or food is similarly limited. In addition, calcium competes with magnesium for absorption, so you need to avoid supplements that combine the two. Absorbable forms of oral magnesium include magnesium chloride, magnesium citrate, magnesium malate, magnesium ascorbate, and others, often described as chelated magnesium. The dose should be split and taken several times a day. For example, to obtain about 400 milligrams of magnesium, take 100 milligrams four times a day with meals. Check the container to ensure that the tablets actually contain this weight of magnesium metal (Mg). People on limited budgets sometimes choose to take food or pharmaceutical grade magnesium sulfate powder, which is available in bulk. Magnesium supplements may help you relax, improve your mood, provide additional energy, and generally benefit your health.

Magnesium supplementation should not be confused with calcium supplementation: a person with atherosclerosis is far more likely to be deficient in magnesium. By contrast, abnormal calcium biochemistry is characteristic of atherosclerosis, along with calcium deposits in the arterial wall. We do not recommend calcium supplements, which make magnesium uptake more difficult. Furthermore, a recent study suggested calcium supplements should be avoided because of increased risk of heart attack.[11] However, despite this media hype, the reported risk from calcium is relatively small and the result has almost no relevance to an individual. In any event, supplemental magnesium will help normalize calcium in the body, as will vitamins D and K.

#6   Alpha-Lipoic Acid

Alpha-lipoic acid is a small, mobile antioxidant, which is soluble in both water and oil. It supports many of the effects of vitamin C. Because of its chemical properties, we would expect this substance to enter arterial plaques. It is a powerful antioxidant and may provide protection against heart disease.[12] Alpha-lipoic acid forms part of the antioxidant network and can chemically reduce other antioxidants by donating electrons to them. This allows it to enhance the functions of vitamin C and to act as a substitute for vitamin E.[13]

A study of the Japanese quail showed that alpha-lipoic acid has a preventive effect on the development of arterial plaques.[14] This little bird (*Coturnix coturnix japonica*) may be a useful laboratory animal for the study of atherosclerosis, as it is omnivorous and easy to maintain. It is also susceptible to both spontaneous and cholesterol-induced atherosclerosis. Some birds have a reduced capability for making vitamin C. While it is not an essential nutrient for the quail, supplementation reduces the requirement for the antioxidant riboflavin (vitamin B2) by half,[15] so the bird may make use of vitamin C in the diet. Like humans, Japanese quail develop plaques in their aortas and sometimes in their coronary arteries; slow-release alpha-lipoic acid inhibits the development of such plaques.

Alpha-lipoic acid has a strong anti-inflammatory action on damaged arterial walls[16] and stimulates production of nitric oxide, which signals the artery walls to relax. Taken together with vitamin C, alpha-lipoic acid improves vasodilatation in the arteries of diabetics.[17] In rats that have consumed high levels of cholesterol and developed atherosclerosis, alpha-lipoic acid reduces the size of the plaques, prevents oxidation, and damps down inflammation.[18] Similar results have been reported in rabbits,[19] and in mice.[20]

In humans, alpha-lipoic acid changes the composition of blood fats in a way that suggests it could provide protection from heart disease.[21] It inhibits the attraction of white blood cells to inflamed tissues more powerfully than aspirin,[22] thus hindering one of the first steps in plaque formation—the adhesion of white blood cells to the arterial wall.[23] The anti-inflammatory effect of alpha-lipoic acid may result from its antioxidant activity,[24] as well as by modifying gene expression.[25]

Alpha-lipoic acid is generally considered a safe food supplement. Since the aim is to generate a reducing (antioxidant) state inside plaque tissues, the addition of alpha-lipoic acid to the diet is justified. In the region of 100–200 milligrams a day of R-alpha-lipoic acid might be appropriate for prevention of heart disease and stroke, and up to 600 milligrams a day for people hoping to reverse the established disease. In each case, it is better to split the intake into three smaller doses, to be taken with meals.

#7   Glycosaminoglycans

We have seen how chondroitin appears to play a protective role in atherosclerosis and may even reverse the disease. Chondroitin is one of several molecules called glycosaminoglycans. It is often combined in supplements with hyaluronic acid or glucosamine. These substances are involved in strengthening and supporting our bodies, and in wound healing. The benefit of these supplements is easily understood, since arterial stress, ineffective healing, and subsequent chronic inflammation are causative in atherosclerosis.

Large doses of chondroitin sulfate may reverse chronic atherosclerosis. Dr. Lester Morrison gave his heart patients several grams of chondroitin sulfate each day and reported outstanding results. In arteries that have been chronically inflamed for years, there is likely to be some residual damage and scarring. However, Morrison's reports suggest that chondroitin may stabilize the condition and remove the immediate risk of heart attack or stroke.

For people who are at high-risk of atherosclerosis, chondroitin sulfate, glucosamine, and hyaluronic acid would be a suitable combination for supplementation. These might be combined with high intakes of vitamins B and C. In the absence of full clinical trials, an intake of several grams of chondroitin (say, 3,000–6,000 milligrams), and reasonable intakes of glucosamine (1,500 milligrams) and hyaluronic acid (200 milligrams), combined with similar or larger intakes of vitamin C, may be an effective nutritional treatment.

#8   Resveratrol

The "French paradox" is a common phrase that is used to express the low levels of atherosclerosis in the country's population, despite the presence of risk factors. French food has high levels of saturated fat and low levels of vegetable oil, compared with that in the United States.[26] The popular press and conventional medicine have suggested that the French have lower rates of coronary disease because they drink more alcohol—in particular, red wine. This is a very nice idea, but probably reflects rather wishful thinking. By all means, drink and enjoy the occasional glass of wine, but beware the irrational expectation that alcohol will prevent a heart attack. There are excellent reasons to explain why people in the U.S. have higher rates of cardiovascular disease than the French. To understand the issue, we need to look more closely at the French diet.

Smoking is more common in France than in the U.S., but the difference is not sufficient to produce higher levels of coronary disease. The French eat more fish, providing higher levels of omega-3 fatty acids,[27] which inhibit inflammation and abnormal blood clotting. Additionally, the French diet has smaller portions and contains less sugar, which would help them avoid atherosclerosis.

The saturated fat content in the French diet is largely irrelevant: clearly, it does not increase the overall incidence of heart attack! The French paradox exists only because of the suggestion that risk factors such as saturated fat should cause French people to have high rates of heart disease. The realization that saturated fat and cholesterol do not cause the disease removes the paradox. Their lower intake of sugar, together with increased amounts of fish and olive oils, is protective.

The French diet also contains higher levels of resveratrol and other antioxidants. Red wine and the skin of grapes contain small amounts of resveratrol, a potent antioxidant, anti-inflammatory, cancer preventative, and anti-aging substance.[28] Given its anti-inflammatory[29] and antioxidant properties, it might be expected to prevent atherosclerosis. Resveratrol and olive oil in the French diet help maintain the lining of the blood vessels, protecting against damage and inflammation.[30] The substance also protects muscle cells in the arterial wall,[31] promotes nitric oxide release,[32] and prevents abnormal blood clotting.[33]

From experimental studies, resveratrol would appear to be an excellent supplement for preventing heart disease. However, as with most effective nutrients, there have been several attempts to demonstrate that it does not work. It has been claimed that resveratrol supplements are not absorbed, are rapidly broken down,[34] or are eliminated from the body. The claimed result is that it is not available and can have no effect in the body. [35] On the other hand, a competent biochemist could surmise that the tissues of the body may regenerate resveratrol from its absorbed metabolites and provide the beneficial effects. Clinical trials on resveratrol are underway and the results are eagerly awaited.

One report suggests that resveratrol is both absorbed and beneficial in humans; it concerns the vision of an 80-year-old man, with night driving problems.[36] The light-sensitive retina at the back of the eye is often examined during an eye test, to give an indication of the health of the small blood vessels, some of which are visible in the retina. As we age, lipofuscin, a yellow-brown granular pigment, is deposited in our cells; these deposits are also visible in the retina. In effect, we can examine the back of the eye to check on the aging of our bodies, particularly the blood vessels. Lipofuscin can be removed from cells in culture and in animal models using antioxidants and substances that remove free iron.

The old man with impaired vision had deposits of lipofuscin in his retina. He was given a supplement containing resveratrol and was rechecked five months later. All his measures of visual function had improved and the lipofuscin was clearing. He also reported that his mental functioning had improved. This appears to be the first report of lipofuscin reversal in the human eye using nutritional supplementation. More importantly, it shows that resveratrol supplements may have an effect in humans and that the objections to its use may be misguided.

Supplements of resveratrol are available and are considered safe. It may be useful in prevention and treatment of atherosclerosis and heart disease. People with no specific indication or risk of atherosclerosis may elect to wait until the results of studies on humans become available. Those with existing or progressive disease might choose to supplement with resveratrol, on the grounds that the risk of waiting exceeds the risk of wasting the supplement cost. Note that numerous other benefits are reported in experiments and animal testing. Supplementing up to three times a day with 250 milligrams of trans-resveratrol, or equivalent, is appropriate.

#9   Fish Oil

Even mainstream medicine suggests that oily fish may help prevent heart disease. To some, this may be comforting, as it has the official stamp of approval; others may regard such endorsement with caution. Their reasoning goes something like this: corporate medicine has the problem that its products are often ineffective, so if oily fish really were helpful, they might not be studied or promoted. Notably, official recommendations suggest people get their fish oil from fish, rather than supplements. This is a mistake: the cardiovascular benefits of fish arise largely from the oils they contain, so a concentrated fish oil supplement is preferable, especially for daily consumption.

In moderation, fish is a wonderful food and one we very much enjoy. However, we would caution against regarding fish itself as a medicine. Although fish contain health-giving oils, they can also accumulate toxic pollutants such as mercury in their flesh. The Mad Hatter in Lewis Carroll's *Alice in Wonderland* stories was inspired by the phrase "as mad as a hatter," which, in turn, was inspired by the mercury poisoning that commonly afflicted hat makers (mercury was used in making felt for hats). Unfortunately, mercury is a brain poison and its symptoms are less amusing than Lewis Carroll's creation. Today, a major source of mercury poisoning is reported to be fish; high-fructose corn syrup and vaccination can also contribute to a person's mercury load.

An infamous case of mercury poisoning occurred in Minamata, Japan. Chisso, a chemical company, had been releasing pollutants since 1908. From 1932 to 1968, methyl mercury was released as an industrial pollutant and accumulated in the shellfish and fish of Minamata Bay. In the mid-1950s, researchers documented an epidemic of neurological problems in the local population. Not only was the illness found in people—their pets and local wild animals were also sick and behaving oddly. The disorder was serious and by 2001, 2,265 local people had been certified as having the disease; another 690 people were diagnosed in the Agano River basin, which was also affected.[37] About three in ten people with the disease died.[38] Fortunately, since the early 1970s, the pollution problem in the area has declined. Sea fish more generally can be contaminated with mercury. Famously, in December 1970, Professor Bruce McDuffie tested a can of tuna fish and raised the alarm.[39] McDuffie found that both tuna and swordfish in his samples were contaminated. The U.S. Food and Drug Administration (FDA) immediately removed a million cans of tuna from the market, as their mercury levels exceeded legal limits.

Whole fish may contain other environmental toxins, such as polychlorinated biphenyls and organochlorine pesticides. The poison levels vary, depending on both the source and the toxin, but both farm-raised and wild fish can be contaminated. Eating polluted fish may negate any beneficial effects of fish on the cardiovascular system. To reduce your intake of contaminants, choose fish from the bottom of the food chain, such as sardines, herrings, pollock, crab, or shrimp. Large predator fish, such as shark or albacore tuna, should be consumed less frequently. This is because a predator fish eats lots of smaller fish and the mercury from these is concentrated in its body—ultimately leading to high levels in top level predators.

Fortunately, when fish oil is extracted for use in supplements, the toxins are removed. Fish oils thus provide benefits to the cardiovascular system without the risk of toxicity.[40] Despite this, corporate medicine suggests eating fish rather than supplements. We hope the reader will use their own judgment. The level of contamination in fish is not sufficient to avoid occasional meals of this delicious food. However, with repeated doses for prevention of illness, whole fish may be less effective than fish oil supplements.

An appropriate intake of fish oil to prevent heart disease is 1,000–3,000 milligrams a day. A higher intake may be useful for those with existing disease or who wish to inhibit blood clotting.

#10   Vitamins D$_3$ and K

Vitamin D plays a crucial role in preventing cardiovascular disease. Deficiency is common—about half the population does not even get the minimum requirement.[41] This vitamin is a little different, as people's skin can produce it in large amounts on a sunny day. Sunlight, rather than food, is often the primary source. For this reason, people who live in higher latitudes are more likely to be deficient. However, even those who live in sunny climes, such as South Florida, may not get enough in the winter.[42]

Deficiency is widespread, particularly among the elderly and those who spend little time in the sun. It is unlikely that a person gets sufficient vitamin D from food alone; a typical diet contains only modest amounts. The easiest way to get enough vitamin D is by taking supplements. As we were writing, forty cases of full-blown rickets were reported in children from Southampton, an affluent city on the relatively sunny south coast of England. Professor Nicholas Clarke stated that "we're seeing cases reminiscent of the 17th century, which would have been inconceivable a year ago."[43] Tragically, these children are sick—almost a century after the disease was thought to have been cured and made an illness of the past. The experts suggested that computer games and children not playing outside was the cause of modern rickets. We have an alternative explanation: the parents believed the authorities' much repeated claims that people do not need supplements! The use of a good-quality multivitamin would have stopped the children becoming ill with rickets and would potentially have protected them from several more long-term illnesses.

People in the polar regions are more likely to have a heart attack or stroke than those who live nearer the equator; this suggests that lack of vitamin D may be having an effect. The evidence implies that shortage of vitamin D may contribute to cardiovascular disease. Deficiency is linked with a range of chronic illness, including conditions associated with cardiovascular disease, such as inflammation, high blood pressure, kidney disease, and diabetes. Heart attack sufferers typically have low levels of vitamin D. Furthermore, raising vitamin D levels protects against numerous other conditions such as flu, multiple sclerosis, tuberculosis, and cancer, in addition to guarding against bone fractures.

The amount of vitamin D in the blood is critical. Typical advice suggests an optimal blood level of 30–50 ng/mL of 25-hydroxy D, rising to 70–100 ng/mL for those with cardiovascular disease. Increasingly, people are encouraged to have their blood levels measured in order to monitor the effects of supplementation. However, this is likely to be costly and, for most people, taking a high-dose supplement of vitamin D_3 is sufficient health insurance.

The government recommended intakes (RDA) of vitamin D are far too low, in the range of 200–600 IU. Currently, informed opinion suggests an optimal intake for adults of 5,000 IU of vitamin D$_3$ a day, even in summer. Making sure you have an intake at this level should ensure that your blood levels are toward the higher end of the required range. Take vitamin D$_3$ (cholecalciferol), rather than the synthetic form, D2 (ergocalciferol). Also, do not be fooled by purported "high-dose" supplements of up to only 1,000–2,000 IU.

Vitamin D is normally considered as the "strong bones" vitamin, which prevents rickets. Vitamin K is also involved in calcium metabolism and in maintaining a healthy skeleton. Both may combine to regulate calcium handling in the body, helping keep it in the bones rather than being deposited in the arteries. There is good reason to consider that most people are also short of vitamin K, and this deficiency contributes to calcification of the arteries. Those in good health can consider a high-dose supplement (500 mcg a day). However, people with existing cardiovascular disease should consult their physician.

Making sure you have optimal blood levels of vitamins D and K will help prevent and treat coronary disease. Vitamin D will also lower your risk of a range of infectious and chronic diseases, including cancer.

Cautionary note (explained previously): *do not take vitamin K if you are on the drug warfarin.*

IMPORTANT POINTS

- Smoking is a personal choice, which has both health and financial costs.

- Eating less fructose will ensure a healthier diet and prevent chronic disease.

- Nutritional supplements are a low-cost approach to cardiovascular disease.

- Taking control of nutrition means a healthier, longer, and more productive life.

- Good health is the natural state and does not need to cost a fortune.

DEMAND
GOOD HEALTH

Heart attack and stroke are not an inevitable part of adult life. Some people live to an old age with healthy cardiovascular systems. Similarly, animals generally do not suffer the same forms of atherosclerosis as humans. The primary difference seems to be in the level of available antioxidants. Most animals synthesize vitamin C in huge amounts, but humans, other primates, guinea pigs, and a few other diverse species have lost the ability to manufacture their own vitamin C and need to get it from the diet. Strangely, humans are officially assumed to need very little vitamin C, far less than even monkeys or guinea pigs in captivity. Vitamin C deficiency may be the main reason so many people are dying prematurely of heart disease and stroke.

Forget about statistical risk factors for atherosclerosis—we need to understand the physiological mechanisms. A dynamic flow of vitamin C can provide sufficient antioxidants to quench the oxidation involved in damage to the arteries and can stem the resultant chronic inflammation. Individual people need different amounts of vitamin C, but at least 3 grams a day would be required for a healthy adult to achieve dynamic flow. Smoking is a "risk factor" because it pollutes the tissues with free radicals, destroys vitamin C, and promotes inflammation.

Remove fructose from your diet: it enlarges the liver, makes people fat around the waist, damages the arteries, and produces the lipid profile considered so dangerous by mainstream medicine.

Fructose is contained in sugar (sucrose) and, particularly, high-fructose corn syrup. There are other ways of sweetening food that are less dangerous: those with a sweet tooth could use glucose, or a natural sweetener, such as stevia. If you fear atherosclerosis, then be sure to avoid fructose.

We have provided a list of simple ways to change your diet to prevent or reverse heart disease. For those wanting to prevent the disease, we suggest small steps. Try one supplement at a time and see how it makes you feel. Lower your sugar intake gradually—perhaps start by having less in your coffee or tea. Make sure what you are doing is sustainable. If you find it almost impossible to come off junk food, then at least take dynamic flow vitamin C and a good multivitamin. The cost is low and the benefit could be ten or twenty extra years of productive life.

Those who already have atherosclerosis or a related condition such as diabetes, or who have had a heart attack or stroke, probably do not need encouragement to get back to good health. The illness may be stabilized by taking dynamic flow vitamin C and other antioxidant supplements, which may lower the risk of another event. However, reversal of atherosclerosis needs more effort and higher levels of antioxidants.

The intake of vitamin C required to reverse the disease is probably in excess of 10 grams a day, preferably including some liposomal vitamin C. The tocotrienol form of vitamin E may also be effective. Alpha-lipoic acid would work well with either or both of these antioxidants. Reversing the disease is far more difficult than preventing the problem in the first place. Despite this, the limited evidence available indicates that atherosclerosis can be reversed with supplements. By making relatively small changes to your lifestyle, you can take back your life and stop being afraid of heart disease.

REFERENCES

Chapter 1: The Number One Killer

1. World Health Organization (WHO). (2009) "Cardiovascular Diseases (CVDs)." World Health Organization Fact Sheet No. 317. Geneva: WHO, 2009.

2. Jackson, G. *Heart Health*. London: Class Publishing, 2000.

3. Cutting, D. *Stop That Heart Attack*. London: Class Publishing, 2001.

4. Scribner, A.W., J. Loscalzo, C. Napoli. "The Effect of Angiotensin-converting Enzyme Inhibition on Endothelial Function and Oxidant Stress." *Eur J Pharmacol* 482 (2003): 95–99. Elisaf, M. "Effects of Fibrates on Serum Metabolic Parameters." *Curr Med Res Opin* 18 (2002): 269–276. Vane, J.R., and R.M. Botting. "The Mechanism of Action of Aspirin." *Thromb Res* 110 (2003): 255–258. Carneado, J., M. Alvarez de Sotomayor, C. Perez-Guerrero, et al. "Simvastatin Improves Endothelial Function in Spontaneously Hypertensive Rats Through a Superoxide Dismutase Mediated Antioxidant Effect." *J Hypertens* 20 (2002): 429–437. Erkkila, L., M. Jauhiainen, K. Laitinen, et al. "Effect of Simvastatin, an Established Lipid-lowering Drug, on Pulmonary *Chlamydia pneumoniae* Infection in Mice." *Antimicrob Agents Chemother* 49:9 (2005): 3959–3962.

5. Weber, C., E. Wolfgang, K. Weber, P.C. Weber. "Increased Adhesiveness of Isolated Monocytes to Epithelium is Prevented by Vitamin C Intake in Smokers." *Circulation* 93 (1996): 1488–1492.

Chapter 2 : The Heart and Cardiovascular System

1. Hasleton, P.S. "The Internal Surface Area of the Adult Human Lung." *J Anat* 112:Pt 3 (1972): 391–400.

2. Rawlins, L., M. Woollard, J. Williams, P. Hallam. "Effect of Listening to 'Nellie the Elephant' During CPR Training on Performance of Chest Compressions by Lay People: Randomised Crossover Trial." *Br Med J* 339 (2009): b4707.

3. Salzar, R.S., M.J. Thubrikar, R.T. Eppink. "Pressure-induced Mechanical Stress in the Carotid Artery Bifurcation: A Possible Correlation to Atherosclerosis." *J Biomech* 28:11 (1995): 1333–1340.

4. Ford, B.J. "Revealing the Ingenuity of the Living Cell." *Biologist* 53:4 (2006): 221–224.

5. Hickey, D.S., and L.A. Noriega. "Relationship Between Structure and Information Processing in *Physarum polycephalum*." *Int J Model Identif Control* 4:4 (2008): 348–356.

Chapter 3: Atherosclerosis

1. Navab, M., J.A. Berliner, A.D. Watson, et al. "The Yin and Yang of Oxidation in the Development of the Fatty Streak. A Review Based on the 1994 George Lyman Duff Memorial Lecture." *Arterioscler Thromb Vasc Biol* 16:7 (1996): 831–842.

2. Clare, K., S.J. Hardwick, K.L. Carpenter, et al. "Toxicity of Oxysterols to Human Monocyte-macrophages." *Atherosclerosis* 118:1 (1995): 67–75.

3. Parhami, F., A.D. Morrow, J. Balucan, et al. "Lipid Oxidation Products Have Opposite Effects on Calcifying Vascular Cell and Bone Cell Differentiation. A Possible Explanation for the Paradox of Arterial Calcification in Osteoporotic Patients." *Arterioscler Thromb Vasc Biol* 17:4 (1997): 680–687.

4. Parthasarathy, S., D. Steinberg, J.L. Witztum. "The Role of Oxidized Low-density Lipoproteins in the Pathogenesis of Atherosclerosis." *Annu Rev Med* 43 (1992): 219–225.

5. Han, D.K., C.C. Haudenschild, M.K. Hong, et al. "Evidence for Apoptosis in Human Atherogenesis and in a Rat Vascular Injury Model." *Am J Pathol* 147:2 (1995): 267–277.

6. Darley-Usmar, V., and B. Halliwell. "Blood Radicals." *Pharm Res* 13 (1996): 649–662.

7. Halpert, I., U.I. Sires, J.D. Roby, et al. "Matrilysin is Expressed by Lipid-laden Macrophages at Sites of Potential Rupture in Atherosclerotic Lesions and Localizes to Areas of Versican Deposition, a Proteoglycan Substrate for the Enzyme." *Proc Natl Acad Sci U S A* 93:18 (1996): 9748–9753.

8. Gieseg, S.P., D.S. Leake, E.M. Flavall, et al. "Macrophage Antioxidant Protection Within Atherosclerotic Plaques." *Front Biosci* 14 (2009): 1230–1246.

9. van der Wal, A.C., O.J. de Boer, A.E. Becker. "Pathology of Acute Coronary Syndromes." In: Parnham, M.J. (ed.). *Progress in Inflammation Research*. Basel: Birkhäuser Verlag, 2001.

10. Dandona, P., A. Aljada, A. Chaudhuri. "Vascular Reactivity and Thiazolidinediones." *Am J Med* 115 (2003): 81S–86S.

11. Williams, B. "Mechanical Influences on Vascular Smooth Muscle Cell Function." *J Hypertens* 16 (1998): 1921–1929. Thorin, E., and S.M. Shreeve. "Heterogeneity of Vascular Endothelial Cells in Normal and Disease States." *Pharmacol Ther* 78 (1998): 155–166. Lindop, G.B., J.J. Boyle, P. McEwan, C.J. Kenyon. "Vascular Structure, Smooth Muscle Cell Phenotype and Growth in Hypertension." *J Hum Hypertens* 9 (1995): 475–478.

12. Watanabe, T., R. Pakala, T. Katagiri, C.R. Benedict. "Monocyte Chemotactic Protein 1 Amplifies Serotonin-induced Vascular Smooth Muscle Cell Proliferation." *J Vasc Res* 38 (2001): 341–349. Rainger, G.E., and G.B. Nash. "Cellular Pathology of Atherosclerosis: Smooth Muscle Cells Prime Cocultured Endothelial Cells for Enhanced Leukocyte Adhesion." *Circ Res* 88 (2001): 615–622. Desai, A., H.A. Lankford, J.S. Warren. "Homocysteine Augments Cytokine-induced Chemokine Expression in Human Vascular Smooth Muscle Cells: Implications for Atherogenesis." *Inflammation* 25 (2001): 179–186.

13. Libby, P. "Changing Concepts of Atherogenesis." *J Intern Med* 247 (2000): 349–358.

14. Kockx, M.M., and A.G. Herman. "Apoptosis in Atherosclerosis: Beneficial or Detrimental?" *Cardiovasc Res* 45 (2000): 736–746. Gronholdt, M.L., S. Dalager-Pedersen, E. Falk. "Coronary Atherosclerosis: Determinants of Plaque Rupture." *Eur Heart J* 19 (1998): C24–C29.

15. Bennett, M.R. "Breaking the Plaque: Evidence for Plaque Rupture in Animal Models

of Atherosclerosis." *Arterioscler Thromb Vasc Biol* 22 (2002): 713–714. Bennett, M.R. "Vascular Smooth Muscle Cell Apoptosis—A Dangerous Phenomenon in Vascular Disease." *J Clin Basic Cardiol* 3 (2000): 63–65.

16. Libby, P. "Atherosclerosis: The New View." *Sci Am* (May 2002): 29–37. Virmani, R., F.D. Kolodgie, A.P. Burke, A. Farb. "Inflammation in Coronary Atherosclerosis—Pathological Aspects." In: Parnham, M.J. (ed.). *Progress in Inflammation Research*. Basel: Birkhäuser Verlag, 2001. Schieffer, B., and H. Drexler. "Role of Interleukins in Relation to the Renin-angiotensin-system in Atherosclerosis." In: Parnham, M.J. (ed.). *Progress in Inflammation Research*. Basel: Birkhäuser Verlag, 2001.

17. Schmitz, G., and M. Torzewski. "Atherosclerosis: An Inflammatory Disease." In: Parnham, M.J. (ed.). *Progress in Inflammation Research*. Basel: Birkhäuser Verlag, 2001.

18. Morrow, D.A., and P.M. Ridker. "C-reactive Protein—A Prognostic Marker of Inflammation in Atherosclerosis." In: Parnham, M.J. (ed.). *Progress in Inflammation Research*. Basel: Birkhäuser Verlag, 2001. Rader, D.J. "Inflammatory Markers of Coronary Risk." *N Engl J Med* 343:16 (October 2000): 1179–1182.

19. Shovman, O., Y. Levy, B. Gilburd, Y. Shoenfeld. "Anti-inflammatory and Immunomodulatory Properties of Statins." *Immunol Res* 25:3 (2002): 271–285. Blake, G.J., and P.M. Ridker. "Are Statins Anti-inflammatory?" *Curr Control Trials Cardiovasc Med* 1 (2000): 161–165. Sukhova, G.K., J.K. Williams, P. Libby. "Statins Reduce Inflammation in Atheroma of Nonhuman Primates Independent of Effects on Serum Cholesterol." *Arterioscler Thromb Vasc Biol* 22:9 (2002): 1452–1458.

20. Aikawa, M., S. Sugiyama, C.C. Hill, et al. "Lipid Lowering Reduces Oxidative Stress and Endothelial Cell Activation in Rabbit Atheroma." *Circulation* 106:11 (2002): 1390–1396.

21. Kooyenga, D.K., M. Geller, T.R. Watkins, M.L. Bierenbaum. "Antioxidant-induced Regression of Carotid Stenosis Over Three Years." Proceedings of the 16th International Congress of Nutrition, Montreal, Canada, 1997. Witztum, J.L., and D. Steinberg. "Role of Oxidised Low-density Protein in Atherogenesis." *J Clin Invest* 88 (1991): 1785–1792. Jialal, I., and S. Devaraj. "The Role of Oxidised Low-density Lipoprotein in Atherogenesis." *J Nutr* 126 (1996): 1053S–1057S.

22. Souza, H.P., and J.L. Zweier. "Free Radicals as Mediators of Inflammation in Atherosclerosis." In: Parnham, M.J. (ed.). *Progress in Inflammation Research*. Basel: Birkhäuser Verlag, 2001.

23. Young, S., and J. McEneny. "Lipoprotein Oxidation and Atherosclerosis." *Biochem Soc Trans* 29:2 (2001): 358–361. Napoli, C., and L.O. Lerman. "Involvement of Oxidation-Sensitive Mechanisms in the Cardiovascular Effects of Hypercholesterolaemia." *Mayo Clin Proc* 76 (2001): 619–631.

24. Frei, B., R. Stocker, B.N. Ames. "Antioxidant Defences and Lipid Peroxidation in Blood Plasma." *Proc Natl Acad Sci U S A* 85 (1988): 9748–9752. Jialal, I., G.L. Vega, S.M. Grundy. "Physiological Levels of Ascorbate Inhibit the Oxidative Modification of Low-density Lipoprotein." *Atherosclerosis* 82 (1990): 185–191.

25. Frei, B., L. England, B.N. Ames. "Ascorbate is an Outstanding Antioxidant in Human Blood Plasma." *Proc Natl Acad Sci U S A* 86 (1989): 6377–6381.

26. Loscalzo, J. "The Oxidant Stress of Hyperhomocysteinemia." *J Clin Invest* 98 (1996): 5.

27. Dudman, N.P., D.E. Wilcken, R. Stocker. "Circulating Lipid Hydroperoxide Levels in Human Hyperhomocysteinemia: Relevance to Development of Arteriosclerosis." *Arterioscler Thromb* 13:4 (1993): 512–516.

28. American Heart Association, www.americanheart.org. Website accessed August 19, 2006.

29. Das, U.N. "Folic Acid Says NO to Vascular Diseases." *Nutrition* 19 (2003): 686–692.

30. Heitzer, T., C. Brockhoff, B. Mayer, et al. "Tetrahydrobiopterin Improves Endothelium-dependent Vasodilation in Chronic Smokers: Evidence for a Dysfunctional Nitric Oxide Synthase." *Circ Res* 86 (2000): E36–E41. Heller, R., A. Unbehaun, B. Schellenberg, et al. "L-Ascorbic Acid Potentiates Endothelial Nitric Oxide Synthesis Via a Chemical Stabilization of Tetrahydrobiopterin." *J Biol Chem* 276 (2001): 40–47. d'Uscio, L.V., S. Milstien, D. Richardson, et al. "Long-term Vitamin C Treatment Increases Vascular Tetrahydrobiopterin Levels and Nitric Oxide Synthase Activity." *Circ Res* 92 (2003): 88–95.

31. Guilland, J.C., A. Favier, G. Potier de Courcy, et al. "Hyperhomocysteinemia: An Independent Risk Factor or a Simple Marker of Vascular Disease? 1. Basic Data." *Pathol Biol* 51 (2003): 101–110.

32. Yap, S. "Classical Homocystinuria: Vascular Risk and Its Prevention." *J Inherit Metab Dis* 26 (2003): 259–265.

33. Stanger, O., and M. Weger. "Interactions of Homocysteine, Nitric Oxide, Folate and Radicals in the Progressively Damaged Endothelium." *Clin Chem Lab Med* 41 (2003): 1444–1454. Werner-Felmayer, G., G. Golderer, E.R. Werner. "Tetrahydrobiopterin Biosynthesis, Utilization and Pharmacological Effects." *Curr Drug Metab* 3 (2002): 159–173. Creager, M.A., S.J. Gallagher, X.J. Girerd, et al. "L-Arginine Improves Endothelium-dependent Vasodilation in Hypercholesterolemic Humans." *J Clin Invest* 90 (1992): 1248–1253.

34. Garner, B., P.K. Witting, A.R. Waldeck, et al. "Oxidation of High-density Lipoproteins. I. Formation of Methionine Sulfoxide in Apolipoproteins AI and AII is an Early Event that Accompanies Lipid Peroxidation and Can Be Enhanced by Alpha-tocopherol." *J Biol Chem* 273:11 (1998): 6080–6087. Garner, B., A.R. Waldeck, P.K. Witting, et al. "Oxidation of High-density Lipoproteins. II. Evidence for Direct Reduction of Lipid Hydroperoxides by Methionine Residues of Apolipoproteins AI and AII." *J Biol Chem* 273:11 (1998): 6088–6095.

35. Esterbauer, H., G. Wag, H. Puhl. "Lipid Peroxidation and Its Role in Atherosclerosis." *Br Med Bull* 49:3 (1993): 566–576. Esterbauer, H., J. Gebicki, H. Puhl, G. Jurgens. "The Role of Lipid Peroxidation and Antioxidants in Oxidative Modification of LDL." *Free Radic Biol Med* 13:4 (1992): 341–390.

36. Bowry, V.W., D. Mohr, J. Cleary, R. Stocker. "Prevention of Tocopherol-mediated Peroxidation in Ubiquinol-10-free Human Low-density Lipoprotein." *J Biol Chem* 270:11 (1995): 5756–5763.

37. Jialal, I., and S.M. Grundy. "Preservation of Endogenous Antioxidants in Low-density Lipoprotein by Ascorbate But Not Probucol During Oxidative Modification." *J Clin Invest* 87 (1991): 597–601. Scaccini, C., and I. Jialal. "LDL Modification by Activated Polymorphonuclear Leukocytes: A Cellular Model of Mild Oxidative Stress." *Free Rad Biol Med* 16 (1994): 49–55. Carr, A.C., and B. Frei. "Towards a New Recommended Dietary Allowance for Vitamin C Based on Antioxidant and Health Effects in Humans." *Am J Clin Nutr* 69 (1999): 1086, 1087.

38. Martin, A., and B. Frei. "Both Intracellular and Extracellular Vitamin C Inhibit Atherogenic Modification of LDL by Human Vascular Endothelial Cells." *Arterioscler Thromb Vasc Biol* 17:8 (1997): 1583–1590. Gokce, N., and B. Frei. "Basic Research in Antioxidant Inhibition of Steps in Atherogenesis." *J Cardiovasc Risk* 3:4 (1996): 352–357. Jialal, I., and C.J. Fuller. "Effect of Vitamin E, Vitamin C and Beta-carotene on LDL Oxidation and Atherosclerosis." *Can J Cardiol* 11:Suppl G (1995): 97G–103G. Retsky, K.L., and B. Frei. "Vitamin C Prevents Metal Ion–dependent Initiation and Propagation of Lipid Peroxidation in Human Low-density Lipoprotein." *Biochim Biophys Acta* 1257:3 (1995): 279–287. Mezzetti, A., D. Lapenna, S.D. Pierdomenico, et al. "Vitamins E, C and Lipid Peroxidation in Plasma and Arterial Tissue of Smokers and Non-smokers." *Atherosclerosis* 112:1 (1995): 91–99.

39. Benditt, E.P. "Implications of the Monoclonal Character of Human Atherosclerotic Plaques." *Beitr Pathol* 158:4 (1976): 405–416.

40. Pearson, T.A., E.C. Kramer, K. Solez, R.H. Heptinstall. "The Human Atherosclerotic Plaque." *Am J Pathol* 86:3 (1977): 657–664.

41. Penn, A. "Role of Somatic Mutation in Atherosclerosis." *Prog Clin Biol Res* 340C (1990): 93–100.

42. Murry, C.E., C.T. Gipaya, T. Bartosek, et al. "Monoclonality of Smooth Muscle Cells in Human Atherosclerosis." *Am J Pathol* 151:3 (1997): 697–705. Chung, I.M., S.M. Schwartz, C.E. Murry. "Clonal Architecture of Normal and Atherosclerotic Aorta: Implications for Atherogenesis and Vascular Development." *Am J Pathol* 152:4 (1998): 913–923.

43. Andreassi, M.G., N. Botto, M.G. Colombo, et al. "Genetic Instability and Atherosclerosis: Can Somatic Mutations Account for the Development of Cardiovascular Diseases?" *Environ Mol Mutagen* 35:4 (2000): 265–269.

44. Ross, J.S., N.E. Stagliano, M.J. Donovan, et al. "Atherosclerosis: A Cancer of the Blood Vessels?" *Am J Clin Pathol* 116:Suppl (2001): S97–S107.

45. Ross, J.S., N.E. Stagliano, M.J. Donovan, et al. "Atherosclerosis and Cancer: Common Molecular Pathways of Disease Development and Progression." *Ann N Y Acad Sci* 947 (2001): 271–292.

46. Chuang P, Gibney EM, Chan L, Ho PM, Parikh CR. "Predictors of cardiovascular events and associated mortality within two years of kidney transplantation." *Transplant Proc.* 36:5 (2004): 1387–91.

47. Ojo AO. "Cardiovascular complications after renal transplantation and their prevention." *Transplantation.* 15;82:5 (2006): 603–611.

48. Weis, M., and J.P. Cooke. "Cardiac Allograft Vasculopathy and Dysregulation of the NO Synthase Pathway." *Arterioscler Thromb Vasc Biol* 23:4 (2003): 567–575.

49. Moreno, J.M., M.C. Ruiz, N. Ruiz, et al. "Modulation Factors of Oxidative Status in Stable Renal Transplantation." *Transplant Proc* 37:3 (2005): 1428–1430.

Chapter 4: A Big Fat Lie

1. Taubes, G. "What If It's All Been a Big Fat Lie?" *The New York Times* (July 7, 2002).

2. Golier, J.A., P.M. Marzuk, A.C. Leon, et al. "Low Serum Cholesterol Level and Attempted Suicide." *Am J Psychiatry* 152:3 (1995): 419–423.

3. Golomb, B.A., H. Stattin, S. Mednick. "Low Cholesterol and Violent Crime." *J Psychiatr Res* 34:4–5 (2000): 301–309.

4. Ulmer, H., C. Kelleher, G. Diem, H. Concin. "Why Eve is Not Adam: Prospective Follow-up in 149,650 Women and Men of Cholesterol and Other Risk Factors Related to Cardiovascular and All-cause Mortality." *J Womens Health (Larchmt)* 13:1 (2004): 41–53.

5. Schatz, I.J., K. Masaki, K. Yano, et al. "Cholesterol and All-cause Mortality in Elderly People from the Honolulu Heart Program: A Cohort Study." *Lancet* 358:9279 (2001): 351–355.

6. Gordon, B.R., T.S. Parker, D.M. Levine, et al. "Low Lipid Concentrations in Critical Illness: Implications for Preventing and Treating Endotoxemia." *Crit Care Med* 24:4 (1996): 584–589.

7. Gordon, B.R., T.S. Parker, D.M. Levine, et al. "Relationship of Hypolipidemia to Cytokine Concentrations and Outcomes in Critically Ill Surgical Patients." *Crit Care Med* 29:8 (2001): 1563–1568.

8. Ravskow, U. "Is Atherosclerosis Caused by High Cholesterol?" *Q J Med* 95 (2002): 397–403. Ravnskov, U. *The Cholesterol Myths: Exposing the Fallacy That Cholesterol and Saturated Fat Cause Heart Disease.* Winona Lake, IN: New Trends, 2001.

9. Ravnskov, U. *The Cholesterol Myths: Exposing the Fallacy That Cholesterol and Saturated Fat Cause Heart Disease.* Winona Lake, IN: New Trends, 2001. McCully, K., and M. McCully. *The Heart Revolution: The Extraordinary Discovery That Finally Laid the Cholesterol Myth to Rest.* New York: Harper, 2000.

10. Marchand, F. "Ueber Atherosclerosis." Verhandlungen der Kongresse fur Innere Medizin, 21 Kongresse, 1904.

11. Windaus, A. "Ueber der Gehalt Normaler und Atheromastoser Aorten an Cholesterol and Cholesterinester." *Zeitschrift Physiol Chem* 67 (1910): 174.

12. Ignatowski, A.I. "Ueber die Wirkung der Tiershen Einwesses auf der Aorta." *Virchows Arch Pathol Anat* 198 (1909): 248.

13. Anichkov, N., and S. Chalatov. "Ueber Experimentelle Cholester-insteatose: Ihre Bedeutung fur die Enstehung einiger Pathologischer Proessen." *Centrbl Allg Pathol Pathol Anat* 24 (1913): 1–9.

14. Dock, W. "Research in Arteriosclerosis; The First Fifty Years." *Ann Intern Med* 49:3 (1958): 699–705.

15. Mehta, N.J., and I.A. Khan. "Cardiology's 10 Greatest Discoveries of the Twentieth Century." *Tex Heart Inst J* 29:3 (2002): 164–171.

16. Abela GS, Picon PD, Friedl SE, Gebara OC, Miyamoto A, Federman M, Tofler GH, Muller JE. "Triggering of plaque disruption and arterial thrombosis in an atherosclerotic rabbit model." *Circulation* 1;91:3 (1995): 776–784.

17. Cassidy, M. "Coronary Disease: The Harverian Oration." *Lancet* 2 (1946): 587–590.

18. Keys, A. "Recollections of Pioneers in Nutrition: From Starvation to Cholesterol." *J Am Coll Nutr* 9 (1990): 288–291.

19. Keys, A., et al. "The CVD Research Programme of the Laboratory of Physiological Hygiene: The Journal." *Lancet* (1961): 291–295. Keys, A., et al. "Mortality and Coronary Heart Disease among Men Studies for Twenty-three Years." *Arch Intern Med* 128 (1971): 201–214.

20. Keys, A. "From Naples to Seven Countries: A Sentimental Journey." *Prog Biomed Pharmacol* 19 (1983): 130.

21. Keys, A., et al. "Lessons from Serum Cholesterol Studies in Japan, Hawaii and Los Angeles." *Ann Intern Med* (1958): 83–93.

22. Keys, A., et al. "Prediction of Serum Cholesterol Responses of Man to Changes in the Fat in the Diet." *Lancet* 2 (1957): 959–966.

23. Strøm, A., and R.A. Jensen. "Mortality from Circulatory Diseases in Norway 1940–1945." *Lancet* 1 (1951): 126–129. Bang, H.O. "Personal Reflections on Incidence of Ischemic Heart Disease in Oslo During the Second World War." *Acta Med Scand* 210 (1981): 245–248.

24. Enos, W.J., et al. "Coronary Disease Among the United States Soldiers Killed in Action in Korea." *JAMA* 152 (1955): 1090–1093.

25. Pickering, G. "Pathogenesis of Myocardial Infarction." *Br Med J* (February 1964): 517–529.

26. Ad Hoc Committee on Dietary Fat and Atherosclerosis. "Dietary Fat and Its Relation to Heart Attack and Strokes." *Circulation* 23 (1961): 133–136.

27. Bügel, S. "Vitamin K and Bone Health in Adult Humans." *Vitamin Horm* 78 (2008): 393–416.

28. Price, P.A., S.A. Faus, M.K. Williamson. "Warfarin-Induced Artery Calcification Is Accelerated by Growth and Vitamin D." *Arterioscler Thromb Vasc Biol* 20 (2000): 317–327. Danziger, J. "Vitamin K–dependent Proteins, Warfarin, and Vascular Calcification." *Clin J Am Soc Nephrol* 3:5 (2008): 1504–1510.

29. Horton, J.D., and B.M. Bushwick. "Warfarin Therapy: Evolving Strategies in Anticoagulation." *Am Fam Physician* 59:3 (1999): 635–646.

30. Linkins, L.A., P.T. Choi, J.D. Douketis. "Major Bleeding Risk with Warfarin for Deep Vein Thrombosis." *Cleveland Clin J Med* 71:4 (2004): 282.

31. Buckley, M.S., A.D. Goff, W.E. Knapp. "Fish Oil Interaction with Warfarin." *Ann Pharmacother* 38:1 (2004): 50–52.

32. Schwalfenberg, G. "Omega-3 Fatty Acids: Their Beneficial Role in Cardiovascular Health." *Can Fam Physician* 52 (2006): 734–740.

33. Anonymous. "Ask the Doctor. 'I Have Read Good News About Nattokinase and Would Like to Use It to Keep My Blood Thin. Is It a Good Substitute for Aspirin?'" *Heart Advisor* 10:4 (2007): 8.

34. Sumi, H., H. Hamada, K. Nakanishi, H. Hiratani. "Enhancement of the Fibrinolytic Activity in Plasma by Oral Administration of Nattokinase." *Acta Haematol* 84:3 (1990): 139–143.

35. Cesarone, M.R., G. Belcaro, A.N. Nicolaides, et al. "Prevention of Venous Thrombosis in Long-haul Flights with Flite Tabs: The LONFLIT-FLITE Randomized, Controlled Trial." *Angiology* 54:5 (2003): 531–539.

36. Chang, Y.Y., J.S. Liu, S.L. Lai, et al. "Cerebellar Hemorrhage Provoked by Combined Use of Nattokinase and Aspirin in a Patient with Cerebral Microbleeds." *Intern Med* 47:5 (2008): 467–469.

37. Dinehart, S.M., and L. Henry. "Dietary Supplements: Altered Coagulation and Effects on Bruising." *Dermatol-Surg* 31:7 Part 2 (2005): 819–826.

38. McMichael, J. "Anticoagulants: Another View." *Br Med J* (October 1964): 1007.

39. Pickering, G., et al. "An Assessment of Long-term Anticoagulant Administration After Cardiac Infarction." *Br Med J* (October 1964): 837–843.

40. Mitchell, J.R.A. "Come Back Anticoagulants, All May Yet Be Forgiven." In: Jewell, D. (ed.). *Advance Medicine*, Vol. 17. London: Pitman Medical, 1981.

41. Robinson, W.S. "Ecological Correlations and the Behavior of Individuals." *Am Sociol Rev* 15:3 (1950): 351–357.

42. Superko, H.R., M. Nejedly, B. Garrett. "Small LDL and Its Clinical Importance as a New CAD Risk Factor: A Female Case Study." *Prog Cardiovasc Nurs* 17:4 (2002): 167–173.

43. Gigerenzer, G., P.M. Todd, ABC Research Group. *Simple Heuristics That Make Us Smart*. New York: Oxford University Press, 2000.

44. Stehbens, W.E. "Coronary Heart Disease, Hypercholesterolaemia, and Atherosclerosis." *Exp Mol Pathol* 70:2 (2001): 103–119. Stehbens, W.E., and M. Martin. "The Vascular Pathology of Familial Hypercholesterolaemia." *Pathology* 23:1 (1991): 54–61.

45. Sijbrands, E.J.G., R.G.J. Westendorp, J.C. Defesche, et al. "Mortality Over Two Centuries in Large Pedigree with Familial Hypercholesterolaemia: Family Tree Mortality Study." *Br Med J* 322 (2001): 1019–1023.

46. Mach, F. "Inflammation is a Crucial Feature of Atherosclerosis and a Potential Target to Reduce Cardiovascular Events." *Handbook Exp Pharmacol* 170 (2005): 697–722.

47. Gaist, D., U. Jeppesen, M. Andersen, et al. "Statins and Risk of Polyneuropathy, A Case-control Study." *Neurology* 58 (2002): 1333–1337.

48. Ghirlanda, G., A. Oradei, A. Manto, et al. "Evidence of Plasma CoQ_{10}-lowering Effect by HMG-CoA Reductase Inhibitors: A Double-blind, Placebo-controlled Study." *J Clin Pharmacol* 33:3 (1993): 226–229.

49. Bell, D.S. "Resolution of Statin-induced Myalgias by Correcting Vitamin D Deficiency." *South Med J* 103:7 (2010): 690–692.

50. Schmidt, H., R. Hennen, A. Keller, et al. "Association of Statin Therapy and Increased Survival in Patients with Multiple Organ Dysfunction Syndrome." *Intensive Care Med* 32:8 (2006): 1248–1251. Varughese, G.I., J.V. Patel, G.Y. Lip, C. Varma. "Novel Concepts of Statin Therapy for Cardiovascular Risk Reduction in Hypertension." *Curr Pharm Des* 12:13 (2006): 1593–1609. Naito, Y., K. Katada, T. Takagi, et al. "Rosuvastatin Reduces Rat Intestinal Ischemia-reperfusion Injury Associated with the Preservation of Endothelial Nitric Oxide Synthase Protein." *World J Gastroenterol* 12:13 (2006): 2024–2030. Terblanche, M., Y. Almog, R.S. Rosenson, et al. "Statins: Panacea for Sepsis?" *Lancet Infect Dis* 6:4 (2006): 242–248.

51. Schoenhagen, P., E.M. Tuzcu, C. Apperson-Hansen, et al. "Determinants of Arterial Wall Remodeling during Lipid-lowering Therapy: Serial Intravascular Ultrasound Observations from the Reversal of Atherosclerosis with Aggressive Lipid Lowering Therapy (REVERSAL) Trial." *Circulation* 113:24 (2006): 2826–2834. Thomas, M.K., D. Narang, R. Lakshmy, et al. "Correlation between Inflammation and Oxidative Stress in Normocholesterolemic Coronary Artery Disease Patients 'On' and 'Off' Atorvastatin for Short Time Intervals." *Cardiovasc Drugs Ther* 20:1 (2006): 37–44.

52. Stoll, L.L., M.L. McCormick, G.M. Denning, N.L. Weintraub. "Antioxidant Effects of Statins." *Drugs Today* 40:12 (2004): 975. Davignon, J., R.F. Jacob, R.P. Mason. "The Antioxidant Effects of Statins." *Coron Artery Dis* 15:5 (2004): 251–258.

53. Ito, M.K., R.L. Talbert, S. Tsimikas. "Statin-associated Pleiotropy: Possible Beneficial Effects Beyond Cholesterol Reduction." *Pharmacotherapy* 26:7 Part 2 (2006): 85S–97S.

54. Editors. "Cholesterol Screening for U.S. Children Could Save Lives." *New Sci* (July 17, 2010).

55. Wu B.J., L. Yan, F. Charlton, et al. "Evidence That Niacin Inhibits Acute Vascular Inflammation and Improves Endothelial Dysfunction Independent of Changes in Plasma Lipids." *Arterioscler Thromb Vasc Biol* 30:5 (2010): 968–975.

56. Alwaili, K., Z. Awan, A. Alshahrani, J. Genest. "High-density Lipoproteins and Cardiovascular Disease: 2010 Update." *Expert Rev Cardiovasc Ther* 8:3 (2010): 413–423.

57. McGovern, M.E. "Taking Aim at HDL-C. Raising Levels to Reduce Cardiovascular Risk." *Postgrad Med* 117:4 (2005): 29–39.

58. Canner, P.L., K.G. Berge, N.K. Wenger, et al. "Fifteen-year Mortality in Coronary Drug Project Patients: Long-term Benefit with Niacin." *J Am Coll Cardiol* 8:6 (1986): 1245–1255.

59. Song, B., and R.A. DeBose-Boyd. "Insig-dependent Ubiquitination and Degradation of 3-Hydroxy-3-methylglutaryl Coenzyme A Reductase Stimulated by Delta- and Gamma-Tocotrienols." *J Biol Chem* 281 (2006): 25054–25061.

60. Ginter, E. "Cholesterol: Vitamin C Controls Its Transformation to Bile Acids." *Science* 179:74 (1973): 702–704. Hallfrisch, J., V.N. Singh, D.C. Muller, et al. "High Plasma Vitamin C Associated with High Plasma HDL- and HDL2 Cholesterol." *Am J Clin Nutr* 60 (1994): 100–105.

61. Ginter, E., P. Bobek, F. Kubec, et al. "Vitamin C in the Control of Hypercholesterolemia in Man." *Int J Vitam Nutr Res Suppl* 23 (1982): 137–152.

62. Crawford, G.P., C.P. Warlow, B. Bennett, et al. "The Effect of Vitamin C supplements on Serum Cholesterol, Coagulation, Fibrinolysis and Platelet Adhesiveness." *Atherosclerosis* 21 (1975): 451–454.

63. Spittle, C.R. "Atherosclerosis and Vitamin C." *Lancet* (1971): 1280–1281.

64. Morin, R.J. "Arterial Cholesterol and Vitamin C." *Lancet* (1972): 594–595.

65. [No author.] "Creating Fat-enriched Foods." *Biologist* 53:4 (2006):176.

66. Halliwell, B., and J.M.C. Gutteridge. *Free Radicals in Biology and Medicine.* New York: Oxford University Press, 1999.

67. Oarada, M., et al. "The Effect of Dietary Lipid Hydroperoxide on Lymphoid Tissue in Mice." *Biochim Biophys Acta* 960 (1988): 229.

68. Tak Yee, A.W., et al. "Absorption and Lymphatic Transport of Peroxidised Lipids by Rat Small Intestine in Vivo: Role of Mucosal GSH." *Am J Physiol* 262 (1992): G99. Stapran, I., et al. "Oxidised Lipids in the Diet are a Source of Oxidize Lipid in Chylomicrons of Human Serum." *Arterioscler Thromb* 14 (1994): 1900. Umeda, Y., et al. "Kinetics and Uptake in Vivo of Oxidatively Modified Lymph Chylomicrons." *Am J Physiol* 268 (1995): G709.

69. Atkins, R. *Dr. Atkins' New Diet Revolution.* New York: Collins, 2002.

70. Forster, H. "Is the Atkins Diet Safe in Respect to Health?" *Fortschr Med* 96:34 (1978): 1697–1702.

71. Rabast, U., H. Kasper, J. Schonborn. "Comparative Studies in Obese Subjects Fed Car-

bohydrate-restricted and High Carbohydrate 1,000-calorie Formula Diets." *Nutr Metab* 22:5 (1978): 269–277. Samaha, F.F., N. Iqbal, P. Seshadri, et al. "A Low-carbohydrate as Compared with a Low-fat Diet in Severe Obesity." *N Engl J Med* 348:21 (2003): 74–81. Foster, G.D., H.R. Wyatt, J.O. Hill, et al. "A Randomized Trial of a Low-carbohydrate Diet for Obesity." *N Engl J Med* 348:21 (2003): 2082–2090. Truby, H., D. Millward, L. Morgan, et al. "A Randomised Controlled Trial of 4 Different Commercial Weight Loss Programmes in the U.K. in Obese Adults: Body Composition Changes Over 6 Months." *Asia Pac J Clin Nutr* 13:Suppl (2004): S146. Truby, H., S. Baic, A. deLooy, et al. "Randomised Controlled Trial of Four Commercial Weight Loss Programmes in the U.K.: Initial Findings from the BBC 'Diet Trials'." *Br Med J* 332:7553 (2006): 1309–1314.

72. Mayor, S. "Researcher Criticised for Comments on the Atkins Diet." *Br Med J* 327 (2003): 414. Astrup, A., T. Meinert Larsen, A. Harper. "Atkins and Other Low-carbohydrate Diets: Hoax or an Effective Tool for Weight Loss?" *Lancet* 364:9437 (2004): 897–899. Kushner, R.F. "Low-carbohydrate Diets, Con: The Mythical Phoenix or Credible Science?" *Nutr Clin Pract* 20:1 (2005): 13–16.

73. Katz, D.L. "Pandemic Obesity and the Contagion of Nutritional Nonsense." *Public Health Rev* 31:1 (2003): 33–44.

74. Acheson, K.J. "Carbohydrate and Weight Control: Where Do We Stand?" *Curr Opin Clin Nutr Metab Care* 7:4 (2004): 485–492. Wood, R.J., J.S. Volek, Y. Liu, et al. "Carbohydrate Restriction Alters Lipoprotein Metabolism by Modifying VLDL, LDL, and HDL Subfraction Distribution and Size in Overweight Men." *J Nutr* 136:2 (2006): 384–389.

75. Wood, R.J., J.S. Volek, S.R. Davis, et al. "Effects of a Carbohydrate-restricted Diet on Emerging Plasma Markers for Cardiovascular Disease." *Nutr Metab (Lond)* 3:1 (2006): 19.

76. Thomson, J.E., I.N. Scobie, F. Ballantyne, et al. "Effect of Carbohydrate Restriction on Lipoprotein Abnormalities in Maturity-onset Diabetes Mellitus." *Acta Diabetol Lat* 17:1 (1980): 33–39.

77. United States Department of Agriculture. "Dietary Guidelines for Americans 2005." Bethesda, MD: U.S. Department of Agriculture, 2005.

78. Ungar, P.S., and M.F. Teaford. *Human Diet: Its Origin and Evolution.* New York: Praeger, 2002.

79. Volek, J.S., M.J. Sharman, D.M. Love, et al. "Body Composition and Hormonal Responses to a Carbohydrate-restricted Diet." *Metabolism* 51:7 (2002): 864–870. McAuley, K.A., C.M. Hopkins, K.J. Smith, et al. "Comparison of High-fat and High-protein Diets with a High-carbohydrate Diet in Insulin-resistant Obese Women." *Diabetologia* 48:1 (2005): 8–16.

80. Arora, S.K., and S.I. McFarlane. "The Case for Low-carbohydrate Diets in Diabetes Management." *Nutr Metab* 2 (2005): 16.Bloch, A.S. "Low-carbohydrate Diets, Pro: Time to Rethink Our Current Strategies." *Nutr Clin Pract* 20:1 (2005): 3–12.

81. Nuttall, F.Q., and M.C. Gannon. "The Metabolic Response to a High-protein, Low-carbohydrate Diet in Men with Type 2 Diabetes Mellitus." *Metabolism* 55:2 (2006): 243–251. Nielsen, J.V., E. Jonsson, A. Ivarsson. "A Low-carbohydrate Diet in Type 1 Diabetes: Clinical Experience—A Brief Report." *Uppsala J Med Sci* 110:3 (2005): 267–273. Kamuren, Z.T., C.G. McPeek, R.A. Sanders, J.B. Watkins 3rd. "Effects of Low-carbohydrate Diet and Pycnogenol Treatment on Retinal Antioxidant Enzymes in Normal and Diabetic Rats." *J Ocul Pharmacol Ther* 22:1 (2006): 10–18.

82. Greene-Finestone, L.S., M.K. Campbell, S.E. Evers, I.A. Gutmanis. "Adolescents' Low-

carbohydrate-density Diets are Related to Poorer Dietary Intakes." *J Am Diet Assoc* 105:11 (2005): 1783–1788.

83. Food and Nutrition Board. *Dietary Reference Intakes for Energy, Carbohydrate, Fiber, Fat, Fatty Acids, Cholesterol, Protein, and Amino Acids (Macronutrients).* Washington, DC: Institute of Medicine, National Academies Press, 2005.

84. Mensink, R.P.M., and M.B. Katan. "Effect of Dietary Trans-fatty Acids on High-density and Low-density Lipoprotein Cholesterol Levels in Healthy Subjects." *N Engl J Med* 323 (1990): 439–445.

85. Ascherrio, A., M.J. Stampher, W.C. Willett. *Trans-fatty Acids and Coronary Heart Disease, Background and Scientific Review.* Cambridge, MA: Harvard University, 1999.

86. Miller, G.D., and P.J. Huth. "Letter from the Dairy Council to FDA." June 18, 2004. Willett, W.C., M.J. Stampfer, J.E. Manson, et al. "Intake of Trans-fatty Acids and Risk of Coronary Heart Disease Among Women." *Lancet* 341 (1993): 581–585. Ascherio, A., C.H. Hennekens, J.E. Buring, et al. "Trans-fatty Acids Intake and Risk of Myocardial Infarction." *Circulation* 89 (1994): 94–101. Pietinen, P., A. Ascherio, P. Korhonen, et al. "Intake of Fatty Acids and Risk of Coronary Heart Disease in a Cohort of Finnish Men. The Alpha-Tocopherol, Beta-Carotene Cancer Prevention Study." *Am J Epidemiol* 145 (1997): 876–887.

87. Willett, W.C., M.J. Stampfer, J.E. Manson, et al. "Intake of Trans-fatty Acids and Risk of Coronary Heart Disease Among Women." *Lancet* 341 (1993): 581–585.

88. Hu, F.B., M.J. Stampfer, J.E. Manson, et al. "Dietary Fat Intake and the Risk of Coronary Heart Disease in Women." *N Engl J Med* 337:21 (1997): 1491–1499.

89. Booyens, J., C.C. Louwrens, I.E. Katzeff. "The Role of Unnatural Dietary Trans and Cis Unsaturated Fatty Acids in the Epidemiology of Coronary Artery Disease." *Med Hypotheses* 25 (1988): 175–182.

90. Willett, W.C., and A. Ascherio. "Trans-fatty Acids: Are the Effects Only Marginal?" *Am J Public Health* 84 (1994): 722–724.

91. Expert Panel on Trans Fatty Acids and Coronary Heart Disease. "Trans-fatty Acids and Coronary Heart Disease Risk." *Am J Clin Nutr* 62 (1995): 655S–708S.

92. Mozaffarian, D., M.B. Katan, A. Ascherio, et al. "Trans-fatty Acids and Cardiovascular Disease." *N Engl J Med* 354:15 (2006): 1601–1613.

93. Mozaffarian, D., and M.J. Stampfer. "Removing Industrial Trans Fat from Foods." *Br Med J* 340 (2010): c1826.

94. Banting, W. *Letter on Corpulence, Addressed to the Public.* New York: Cosimo Classics, 2005.

95. Brillat-Savarin, J.A. *The Physiology of Taste.* Translated from the last Paris edition by Fayette Robinson. Adelaide eBook, 2007.

Chapter 5: Sweet But Deadly

1. Yudkin, J. *Pure White and Deadly: The Problem of Sugar.* London: Davis Poynter, 1972.

2. McDonald, N.C. "Active Transportation to School: Trends Among U.S. Schoolchildren, 1969–2001." *Am J Prevent Med* 32:6 (2007): 509–516.

3. Kim, J., K.E. Peterson, K.S. Scanlon, et al. "Trends in Overweight from 1980 through

2001 among Preschool-Aged Children Enrolled in a Health Maintenance Organization." *Obesity* 14 (2006): 1107–1112.

4. He, K., L. Zhao, M.L. Daviglus, et al.; INTERMAP Cooperative Research Group. "Association of Monosodium Glutamate Intake With Overweight in Chinese Adults: The INTERMAP Study." *Obesity* 16:8 (2008): 1875–1880.

5. Aso, K., and K. Matsuda. "Studies on the Sugars in Apple Juice." *Tohoku J Agricult Res* 2 (1951): 135–139.

6. Karadeniz, F., and A. Eksi. "Sugar Composition of Apple Juices." *J Eur Food Res Tech* 215:2 (2002): 145–148.

7. Bronstein, A.C., D.A. Spyker, L.R. Cantilena, et al. "2006 Annual Report of the American Association of Poison Control Centers' National Poison Data System (NPDS)." *Clin Toxicol* 45:8 (2007): 815–917.

8. Kritchevsky, D. "The Effects of Feeding Various Carbohydrates on the Development of Hypercholesterolemia and Atherosclerosis." *Adv Exp Med Biol* 60 (1975): 231–249.

9. Yudkin, J. *Pure White and Deadly: The Problem of Sugar.* London: Davis Poynter, 1972.

10. Davies, L. "Obituary: John Yudkin." *Independent* (July 25, 1995).

11. Suzuki, M., D. Yamamoto, T. Suzuki, et al. "Effect of Fructose-rich High-fat Diet on Glucose Sensitivity and Atherosclerosis in Nonhuman Primate." *Methods Find Exp Clin Pharmacol* 28:9 (2006): 609–617.

12. Merat, S., F. Casanada, M. Sutphin, et al. "Western-type Diets Induce Insulin Resistance and Hyperinsulinemia in LDL Receptor-deficient Mice But Do Not Increase Aortic Atherosclerosis Compared with Normoinsulinemic Mice in Which Similar Plasma Cholesterol Levels are Achieved by a Fructose-rich Diet." *Arterioscler Thromb Vasc Biol* 19:5 (1999): 1223–1230.

13. Story, J.A. "Dietary Carbohydrate and Atherosclerosis." *Fed Proc* 41:11 (1982): 2797–2800.

14. Levine, R. "Monosaccharides in Health and Disease." *Annu Rev Nutr* 6 (1986): 211–224.

15. Kohen-Avramoglu, R., A. Theriault, K. Adeli. "Emergence of the Metabolic Syndrome in Childhood: An Epidemiological Overview and Mechanistic Link to Dyslipidemia." *Clin Biochem* 36:6 (2003): 413–420.

16. Tokita, Y., Y. Hirayama, A. Sekikawa, et al. "Fructose Ingestion Enhances Atherosclerosis and Deposition of Advanced Glycated End-products in Cholesterol-fed Rabbits." *J Atheroscler Thromb* 12:5 (2005): 260–267.

17. Gaby, A.R. "Adverse Effects of Dietary Fructose." *Altern Med Rev* 10:4 (2005): 294–306.

18. Bocarsly, M.E., E.S. Powell, N.M. Avena, B.G. Hoebel. (2010) "High-fructose Corn Syrup Causes Characteristics of Obesity in Rats: Increased Body Weight, Body Fat and Triglyceride Levels." *Pharmacol Biochem Behav* 97:1 (November 2010): 101–106.

Chapter 6: Risk Factors and Inflammation

1. Conant, R.C., and W.R. Ashby. "Every Good Regulator of a System Must Be a Model of That System." *Int J Systems Sci* 1:2 (1970): 89–97.

2. Bhaskaran, K., S. Hajat, A. Haines, et al. "Short-term Effects of Temperature on Risk of Myocardial Infarction in England and Wales: Time Series Regression Analysis of the Myocardial Ischaemia National Audit Project (MINAP) Registry." *Br Med J* 341 (2010): c3823.

3. British Medical Journal Group. "Heart Attacks Triggered by Cold Weather, *BMJ* Group." *The Guardian,* guardian.co.uk (August 11, 2010).

4. Le Fanu, J. *The Rise and Fall of Modern Medicine.* London: Little Brown, 1999.

5. Brink, S. "Unlocking the Heart's Secrets." *U.S. News and World Report* 125 (1998): 56–99. Kannel, W.B. "Clinical Misconceptions Dispelled by Epidemiological Research." *Circulation* 92 (1995): 3350–3360.

6. Kannel, W.B., T.R. Dawber, A. Kagan, et al. "Factors of Risk in the Development of Coronary Heart Disease—Six-year Follow-up Experience. The Framingham Study." *Ann Intern Med* 55 (1961): 33–50.

7. Ravnskov, U. "High Cholesterol May Protect Against Infections and Atherosclerosis." *Q J Med* 96 (2003): 927–934.

8. Jacobs, D., H. Blackburn, M. Higgins, et al. "Report of the Conference on Low Blood Cholesterol: Mortality Associations." *Circulation* 86 (1992): 1046–1060.

9. Stehbens, W.E. "Coronary Heart Disease, Hypercholesterolemia, and Atherosclerosis. I. False Premises." *Exp Mol Pathol* 70:2 (2001): 103–119.

10. Ravnskov, U. "Cholesterol Lowering Trials in Coronary Heart Disease: Frequency of Citation and Outcome." *Br Med J* 305 (1992): 5–19.

11. Beaglehole, R., M.A. Foulkes, I.A. Prior, E.F. Eyles. "Cholesterol and Mortality in New Zealand Maoris." *Br Med J* 280 (1980): 285–287.

12. Stehbens, W. "Cholesterol Feeding and Experimental Atherosclerosis." *Atherosclerosis* 73:1 (1988): 85–86.

13. Davies, H. (2010) "*The Daily Mail* List of 'Things That Give You Cancer'." Facebook, http://www.facebook.com/group.php?gid=269512464297; accessed August 16, 2010.

14. Davies, H. "The Second *Daily Mail* List of 'Things That Prevent You From Cancer'." Facebook, http://www.facebook.com/group.php?gid=299519692752; accessed August 16, 2010.

15. Dobson, R. "Can Dogs Give You Breast Cancer? Bizarre Medical Theories That Experts Claim May Actually Be True." *Daily Mail Online* (October 30, 2007); http://www.daily-mail.co.uk/health/article-490581/can-dogs-breast-cancer-bizarre-medical-theories-experts-claim-actually-true.html.

16. Hope, J. "Cats and Dogs Cut Their Owners' Cancer Risk by a Third, Researchers Say." *Daily Mail* (October 8, 2008).

17. Stallones, R.E. "The Rise and Fall of Ischemic Heart Disease." *Sci Am* 243 (2980): 43–49.

18. Harjai, K.J. "Potential New Cardiovascular Risk Factors: Left-ventricular Hypertrophy, Homocysteine, Lipoprotein(a), Triglycerides, Oxidative Stress, and Fibrinogen." *Ann Intern Med* 131 (1999): 376–386. Grant, P.J. "The Genetics of Atherothrombotic Disorders: A Clinician's View." *J Thromb Haemost* 1 (2003): 1381–1390. Maas, R., and R.H. Boger. "Old and New Cardiovascular Risk Factors: From Unresolved Issues to New Opportunities." *Atheroscler Suppl* 4 (2003): 5–17. Dominiczak, M.H. "Risk Factors for Coro-

nary Disease: The Time for a Paradigm Shift?" *Clin Chem Lab Med* 39 (2001): 907–919. Frostegard, J. "Autoimmunity, Oxidized LDL and Cardiovascular Disease." *Autoimmun Rev* 1 (2002): 233–237.

19. Harrison, D.G., H. Cai, U. Landmesser, K.K. Griendling. "Interactions of Angiotensin II with NAD(P)H Oxidase, Oxidant Stress and Cardiovascular Disease." *J Renin Angiotensin Aldosterone Syst* 4 (2003): 51–61. Cuff, C.A., D. Kothapalli, E. Azonobi, et al. "The Adhesion Receptor CD44 Promotes Atherosclerosis by Mediating Inflammatory Cell Recruitment and Vascular Cell Activation." *J Clin Invest* 108 (2001): 1031–1040. Huang, Y., L. Song, S. Wu, et al. "Oxidized LDL Differentially Regulates MMP-1 and TIMP-1 Expression in Vascular Endothelial Cells." *Atherosclerosis* 156 (2001): 119–125. McIntyre, T.M., S.M. Prescott, A.S. Weyrich, G.A. Zimmerman. "Cell–Cell Interactions: Leukocyte-Endothelial Interactions." *Curr Opin Hematol* 10 (2003): 150–158.

20. Gonzalez, M.A., and A.P. Selwyn. "Endothelial Function, Inflammation, and Prognosis in Cardiovascular Disease." *Am J Med* 115 (2003): 99S–106S.

21. Ridker P.M., N. Rifai, L. Rose, et al. "Comparison of C-reactive Protein and Low-density Lipoprotein Cholesterol Levels in the Prediction of First Cardiovascular Events." *N Engl J Med* 347 (2002): 1557–1565. Bermudez, E.A., N. Rifai, J. Buring, et al. "Interrelationships Among Circulating Interleukin-6, C-reactive Protein, and Traditional Cardiovascular Risk Factors in Women." *Arterioscler Thromb Vasc Biol* 22 (2002): 1668–1673. Blake, G.J., and P.M. Ridker. "Inflammatory Biomarkers and Cardiovascular Risk Prediction." *J Intern Med* 252 (2002): 283–294. Pradhan, A.D., N. Rifai, P.M. Ridker, et al. "Soluble Intercellular Adhesion Molecule-1, Soluble Vascular Adhesion Molecule-1, and the Development of Symptomatic Peripheral Arterial Disease in Men." *Circulation* 106 (2002): 820–825.

22. Osiecki, H. "The Role of Chronic Inflammation in Cardiovascular Disease and Its Regulation by Nutrients." *Altern Med Rev* 9:1 (2004): 32–53.

23. Smith, R. "Health Warning Over Statin Taken by Millions." *Daily Telegraph*, telegraph.co.uk (March 20, 2010).

24. Graveline, D., and M. Kendrick. *The Statin Damage Crisis*. Duane Graveline Publishing, 2009. Graveline, D., K.S. McCully, J.S. Cohen. *Lipitor Thief of Memory*. Duane Graveline Publishing, 2006. Graveline, D. *Statin Drugs, Side Effects and the Misguided War on Cholesterol*. Duane Graveline Publishing, 2008.

25. Tilstone, C. "Drug Safety Update." Medicines and Healthcare Products Regulatory Agency 3:4 (2009): 11–12.

26. Bandolier. "Statins." Medicine.ox.ac.uk, 2007; accessed March 30, 2010.

27. Waters, J. "The Other Side of Statins: They've Saved Countless Lives—But Now Doctors Fear for Some, The Side Effects Could Be Devastating." *Daily Mail* (March 30, 2010).

28. Laurance, J. "The A–Z of (Conflicting) Health Advice: We Try to Get to the Bottom of All Those Contradictory Medical Theories." *Daily Mail Online* (November 6, 2009).

29. Macrae, F. "Breakfast Like a King: Why a High-fat Bacon and Eggs Meal is Healthiest Start to the Day (But Only First Thing)." *Daily Mail* (March 31, 2010).

30. Weber, L.J. *Profits Before People? Ethical Standards and the Marketing of Prescription Drugs*. Indianapolis: Indiana University Press, 2006. Henry J. Kaiser Family Foundation. "Views on Prescription Drugs and the Pharmaceutical Industry." *Kaiser Health Report* (January/February 2005); www.kff.org.

Chapter 7: Overlooked Evidence

1. Kaperonis, E.A., C.D. Liapis, J.D. Kakisis, et al. "Inflammation and Atherosclerosis." *Eur J Vasc Endovasc Surg* 31:4 (2006): 386–393.

2. Sardi, B. "The Man Who Cured Heart Disease With a Natural Molecule, 20 Years Before Cholesterol Drugs!" LewRockwell.com; accessed March 28, 2010.

3. Morrison, L.M. *Coronary Heart Disease and the Mucopolysaccharides.* Springfield, IL: Thomas, 1974.

4. Morrison, L., and K. Johnson. "Cholesterol Content of the Coronary Arteries and Blood in Acute Coronary Artery Thrombosis." *Am Heart J* 39:1 (1950): 31–34.

5. Morrison, L.M. "A Nutritional Program for Prolongation of Life in Coronary Atherosclerosis." *JAMA* 159:15 (1955): 1425–1428.

6. Morrison, L., and W.F. Gonzalez. "Results of Treatment of Coronary Arteriosclerosis with Choline." *Am Heart J* 39:5 (1950): 729–736.

7. Morrison, L.M. "Diet in Coronary Atherosclerosis." *JAMA* 173:8 (1960): 884–888.

8. Morrison, L.M., K. Murata, J.J. Quilligan, et al. "Prevention of Atherosclerosis in Subhuman Primates by Chondroitin Sulfate A." *Circ Res* 19:2 (1966): 358–363.

9. Morrison, L.M. "Reduction of Ischemic Coronary Heart Disease by Chondroitin Sulfate A." *Angiology* 22:3 (1971): 165–174.

10. Morrison, L.M., and N. Enrick. "Coronary Heart Disease: Reduction of Death Rate by Chondroitin Sulfate A." *Angiology* 24:5 (1973): 269–287.

11. Morrison, L. (1975) "CSA and CSC in Man and Mammals to Inhibit Atherosclerosis and the Recurrence of Cardiovascular Incidents in Atherosclerotic Mammals." U.S. Patent 3,895,107.

12. Radhakrishnamurthy, B., S.R. Srinivasan, P. Vijayagopal, G.S. Berenson. "Arterial Wall Proteoglycans—Biological Properties Related to Pathogenesis of Atherosclerosis." *Eur Heart J* 11:Suppl E (1990): 148–157.

13. Völker, W., A. Schmidt, W. Oortmann, et al. "Mapping of Proteoglycans in Atherosclerotic Lesions." *Eur Heart J* 11:Suppl E (1990): 29–40.

14. Sobolewski, K., M. Wola?ska, E. Ba?kowski, et al. "Collagen, Elastin and Glycosaminoglycans in Aortic Aneurysms." *Acta Biochim Pol* 42:3 (1995): 301–307.

15. du Souich, P., A.G. García, J. Vergés, E. Montell. "Immunomodulatory and Anti-inflammatory Effects of Chondroitin Sulphate." *J Cell Mol Med* 13:8A (2009): 1451–1463.

16. American Heart Association Nutrition Committee; Lichtenstein, A.H., L.J. Appel, M. Brands, et al. "Diet and Lifestyle Recommendations Revision 2006: A Scientific Statement from the American Heart Association Nutrition Committee." *J Circ* 114:1 (2006): 82–96.

17. Ravnskov, U. *The Cholesterol Myths: Exposing the Fallacy that Saturated Fat and Cholesterol Cause Heart Disease.* Winona Lake, IN: New Trends, 2000.

18. Fyfe, A.I. "Transplant Atherosclerosis: The Clinical Syndrome, Pathogenesis and Possible Model of Spontaneous Atherosclerosis." *Can J Cardiol* 8:5 (1992): 509–519.

19. Vallance, P. "Nitric Oxide." *Biologist* 48 (2001): 153–158. Annuk, M., M. Zilmer, L. Lind, et al. "Oxidative Stress and Endothelial Function in Chronic Renal Failure." *J Am Soc Nephrol* 12 (2001): 2747–2752.

20. D'Orleans-Juste, P., J. Labonte, G. Bkaily, et al. "Function of the Endothelin(B) Receptor in Cardiovascular Physiology and Pathophysiology." *Pharmacol Ther* 95 (2002): 221–238. Annuk, M., M. Zilmer, B. Fellstrom. "Endothelium-dependent Vasodilation and Oxidative Stress in Chronic Renal Failure: Impact on Cardiovascular Disease." *Kidney Int Suppl* 84 (2003): S50–S53. Egashira, K. "Clinical Importance of Endothelial Function in Arteriosclerosis and Ischemic Heart Disease." *Circ J* 66 (2002): 529–533. Luscher, T.F., F.C. Tanner, M.R. Tschudi, G. Noll. "Endothelial Dysfunction in Coronary Artery Disease." *Annu Rev Med* 44 (1993): 395–418.

21. Higgins, J.P. "Can Angiotensin-converting Enzyme Inhibitors Reverse Atherosclerosis?" *South Med J* 96 (2003): 569–579. Harrison, D.G., and H. Cai. "Endothelial Control of Vasomotion and Nitric Oxideproduction." *Cardiol Clin* 21 (2003): 289–302. Stankevicius, E., E. Kevelaitis, E. Vainorius, U. Simonsen. "Role of Nitric Oxide and Other Endothelium-derived Factors." *Medicina (Kaunas)* 39 (2003): 333–341. Vane, J.R., and R.M. Botting. "Secretory Functions of the Vascular Endothelium." *J Physiol Pharmacol* 43 (1992): 195–207. Chauhan, S.D., H. Nilsson, A. Ahluwalia, A.J. Hobbs. "Release of C-type Natriuretic Peptide Accounts for the Biological Activity of Endothelium-derived Hyperpolarizing Factor." *Proc Natl Acad Sci U S A* 100 (2003): 1426–1431.

22. Pearson, J.D. "Endothelial Cell Function and Thrombosis." *Baillieres Best Pract Res Clin Haematol* 12 (1999): 329–341. Huber, D., E.M. Cramer, J.E. Kaufmann, et al. "Tissue-type Plasminogen Activator (t-PA) is Stored in Weibel-Palade Bodies in Human Endothelial Cells Both in Vitro and in Vivo." *Blood* 99 (2002): 3637–3645.

23. Gong, L., G.M. Pitari, S. Schulz, S.A. Waldman. "Nitric Oxide Signaling: Systems Integration of Oxygen Balance in Defense of Cell Integrity." *Curr Opin Hematol* 11 (2004): 7–14. Sumpio, B.E., J.T. Riley, A. Dardik. "Cells in Focus: Endothelial Cell." *Int J Biochem Cell Biol* 34 (2002): 1508–1512. Ando, J., and A. Kamiya. "Blood Flow and Vascular Endothelial Cell Function." *Front Med Biol Engl* 5 (1993): 245–264.

24. Kvasnicka, T. "NO (Nitric Oxide) and Its Significance in Regulation of Vascular Homeostasis." *Vnitr Lek* 49 (2003): 291–296.

25. Lirk, P., G. Hoffmann, J. Rieder. "Inducible Nitric Oxide Synthase—Time for Reappraisal." *Curr Drug Targets Inflamm Allergy* 1 (2002): 89–108. Zhang, J., J. Schmidt, E. Ryschich, et al. "Inducible Nitric Oxide Synthase is Present in Human Abdominal Aortic Aneurysm and Promotes Oxidative Vascular Injury." *J Vasc Surg* 38 (2003): 360–367.

26. Cooke, J.P. "Is Atherosclerosis an Arginine Deficiency Disease?" *J Invest Med* 46 (1998): 377–380.

27. Egashira, K. "Clinical Importance of Endothelial Function in Arteriosclerosis and Ischemic Heart Disease." *Circ J* 66 (2002): 529–533.

28. Tapiero, H., G. Mathe, P. Couvreur, K.D. Tew. "Arginine." *Biomed Pharmacother* 56 (2002): 439–445. Preli, R.B., K.P. Klein, D.M. Herrington. "Vascular Effects of Dietary L-arginine Supplementation." *Atherosclerosis* 162 (2002): 1–15. Tiefenbacher, C.P. "Tetrahydrobiopterin: A Critical Cofactor for eNOS and a Strategy in the Treatment of Endothelial Dysfunction?" *Am J Physiol Heart Circ Physiol* 280 (2001): H2484–H2488.

29. van Hinsbergh, V.W. "NO or H(2)O(2) for Endothelium-dependent Vasorelaxation: Tetrahydrobiopterin Makes the Difference." *Arterioscler Thromb Vasc Biol* 21 (2001): 719–721.

30. Vallance, P., J. Collier, S. Moncada. "Nitric Oxide Synthesised from L-arginine Medi-

ates Endothelium-dependent Dilatation in Human Veins in Vivo." *Cardiovasc Res* 23 (1989): 1053–1057.

31. Vallance, P., J. Collier, S. Moncada. "Effects of Endothelium-derived Nitric Oxide on Peripheral Arteriolar Tone in Man." *Lancet* 2 (1989): 997–1000.

32. Major, T.C., R.W. Overhiser, R.L. Panek. "Evidence for NO Involvement in Regulating Vascular Reactivity in Balloon-injured Rat Carotid Artery." *Am J Physiol* 269 (1995): H988–H996.

33. Cooke, J.P. "Does ADMA Cause Endothelial Dysfunction?" *Arterioscler Thromb Vasc Biol* 20 (2000): 2032–2037. Mukherjee, S., S.D. Coaxum, M. Maleque, S.K. Das. "Effects of Oxidized Low-density Lipoprotein on Nitric Oxide Synthetase and Protein Kinase C Activities in Bovine Endothelial Cells." *Cell Mol Biol* 47 (2001): 1051–1058.

34. Anderson, T.J. "Assessment and Treatment of Endothelial Dysfunction in Humans." *J Am Coll Cardiol* 34 (1999): 631–638. Watts, G.F., D.A. Playford, K.D. Croft, et al. "Coenzyme Q(10) Improves Endothelial Dysfunction of the Brachial Artery in Type II Diabetes Mellitus." *Diabetologia* 45 (2002): 420–426.

35. Hampl, V. "Nitric Oxide and Regulation of Pulmonary Vessels." *Cesk Fysiol* 49 (2000): 22–29.

36. Stankevicius, E., E. Kevelaitis, E. Vainorius, U. Simonsen. "Role of Nitric Oxide and Other Endothelium-derived Factors." *Medicina (Kaunas)* 39 (2003): 333–341.

37. De Nigris, F., L.O. Lerman, W.S. Ignarro, et al. "Beneficial Effects of Antioxidants and L-arginine on Oxidation-sensitive Gene Expression and Endothelial NO Synthase Activity at Sites of Disturbed Shear Stress." *Proc Natl Acad Sci U S A* 100:3 (February 2003): 1420–1425.

38. Cooke, J.P., and R.K. Oka. "Atherogenesis and the Arginine Hypothesis." *Curr Atheroscler Rep* 3 (2001): 252–259.

39. Shmit, E. "Antioxidant Vitamins May Prevent Blood Vessel Blockage and Protect Against Cardiovascular Disease." *UCLA News* (January 15, 2003).

40. Lin, K.Y., A. Ito, T. Asagami, et al. "Impaired Nitric Oxide Synthase Pathway in Diabetes Mellitus: Role of Asymmetric Dimethylarginine and Dimethylarginine Dimethylaminohydrolase." *Circulation* 106 (2002): 987–992. Abbasi, F., T. Asagmi. J.P. Cooke, et al. "Plasma Concentrations of Asymmetric Dimethylarginine are Increased in Patients with Type 2 Diabetes Mellitus." *Am J Cardiol* 88 (2001): 1201–1203. Chan, J.R., R.H. Boger, S.M. Bode-Boger, et al. "Asymmetric Dimethylarginine Increases Mononuclear Cell Adhesiveness in Hypercholesterolemic Humans." *Arterioscler Thromb Vasc Biol* 20 (2000): 1040–1046.

41. Artenie, R., A. Artenie, A. Cosovanu. "The Cardiovascular Significance of Nitric Oxide." *Rev Med Chir Soc Med Nat Iasi* 103 (1999): 48–56. Lyons, D. "Impairment and Restoration of Nitric Oxide-dependent Vasodilation in Cardiovascular Disease." *Int J Cardiol* 62 (1997): S101–S109. Llorens, S., J. Jordan, E. Nava. "The Nitric Oxide Pathway in the Cardiovascular System." *J Physiol Biochem* 58 (2002): 179–188.

42. Verhamme, P., R. Quarck, H. Hao, et al. "Dietary Cholesterol Withdrawal Reduces Vascular Inflammation and Induces Coronary Plaque Stabilization in Miniature Pigs." *Cardiovasc Res* 56 (2002): 135–144.

43. Stuhlinger, M.C., R.K. Oka, E.E. Graf, et al. "Endothelial Dysfunction Induced by Hyperhomocyst(e)inemia: Role of Asymmetric Dimethylarginine." *Circulation* 108 (2003):

933–938. Jonasson, T.F., T. Hedner, B. Hultberg, H. Ohlin. "Hyperhomocysteinaemia is Not Associated with Increased Levels of Asymmetric Dimethylarginine in Patients with Ischaemic Heart Disease." *Eur J Clin Invest* 33 (2003): 543–549.

44. Saitoh, M., T. Osanai, T. Kamada, et al. "High Plasma Level of Asymmetric Dimethylarginine in Patients with Acutely Exacerbated Congestive Heart Failure: Role in Reduction of Plasma Nitric Oxide Level." *Heart Vessels* 18 (2003): 177–182.

45. Rajagopalan, S., D. Pfenninger, C. Kehrer, et al. "Increased Asymmetric Dimethylarginine and Endothelin 1 Levels in Secondary Raynaud's Phenomenon: Implications for Vascular Dysfunction and Progression of Disease." *Arthritis Rheum* 48 (2003): 1992–2000.

46. Heitzer, T., C. Brockhoff, B. Mayer, et al. "Tetrahydrobiopterin Improves Endothelium-dependent Vasodilation in Chronic Smokers: Evidence for a Dysfunctional Nitric Oxide Synthase." *Circ Res* 86 (2000): E36–E41. Ho, F.M., S.H. Liu, C.S. Liau, et al. "High Glucose-induced Apoptosis in Human Endothelial Cells is Mediated by Sequential Activations of c-Jun NH(2)-terminal Kinase and Caspase-3." *Circulation* 101 (2000): 2618–2624. Ho, F.M., S.H. Liu, C.S. Liau, et al. "Nitric Oxide Prevents Apoptosis of Human Endothelial Cells from High Glucose Exposure During Early Stage." *J Cell Biochem* 75 (1999): 258–263.

47. Cooke, J.P. "The Endothelium: A New Target for Therapy." *Vasc Med* 5 (2000): 49–53. Sydow, K., E. Schwedhelm, N. Arakawa, et al. "ADMA and Oxidative Stress are Responsible for Endothelial Dysfunction in Hyperhomocyst(e)inemia: Effects of L-arginine and B Vitamins." *Cardiovasc Res* 57 (2003): 244–252.

48. Werner-Felmayer, G., G. Golderer, E.R. Werner. "Tetrahydrobiopterin Biosynthesis, Utilization and Pharmacological Effects." *Curr Drug Metab* 3 (2002): 159–173.

49. Freedman, J.E., L. Li, R. Sauter, J.F. Kearney Jr. "Alpha-tocopherol and Protein Kinase C Inhibition Enhance Platelet-derived Nitric Oxide release." *FASEB J* 14 (2000): 2377–2379. Jones, W., X. Li, Z.C. Qu, et al. "Uptake, Recycling, and Antioxidant Actions of Alpha-lipoic Acid in Endothelial Cells." *Free Radical Biol Med* 33 (2002): 83–93.

50. Blum, A., R. Porat, U. Rosenschein, et al. "Clinical and Inflammatory Effects of Dietary L-arginine in Patients with Intractable Angina Pectoris." *Am J Cardiol* 83 (1999): 1488–1490.

51. Walker, H.A., E. McGing, I. Fisher, et al. "Endothelium-dependent Vasodilation is Independent of the Plasma L-arginine/ADMA Ratio in Men with Stable Angina: Lack of Effect of Oral L-arginine on Endothelial Function, Oxidative Stress and Exercise Performance." *J Am Coll Cardiol* 38 (2001): 499–505.

52. Ceremuzynski, L., T. Chamiec, K. Herbaczynska-Cedro. "Effect of Supplemental Oral L-arginine on Exercise Capacity in Patients with Stable Angina Pectoris." *Am J Cardiol* 80 (1997): 331–333.

54. Bednarz, B. R. Wolk, T. Chamiek, et al. "Effects of Oral L-arginine Supplementation on Exercise-induced QT Dispersion and Exercise Tolerance in Stable Angina Pectoris." *Int J Cardiol* 75 (2000): 205–210.

54. Egashira, K., Y. Hirooka, T. Kuga, et al. "Effects of L-arginine Supplementation on Endothelium-dependent Coronary Vasodilation in Patients with Angina Pectoris and Normal Coronary Arteriograms." *Circulation* 94 (1996): 130–134.

55. Rector, T.S., A. Bank, K.A. Mullen, et al. "Randomized, Double-blind, Placebo-con-

trolled Study of Supplemental Oral L-arginine in Patients with Heart Failure." *Circulation* 93 (1996): 2135–2141.

56. Watanabe, G., H. Tomiyama, N. Doba. "Effects of Oral Administration of L-arginine on Renal Function in Patients with Heart Failure." *J Hypertens* 18 (2000): 229–234.

57. Schulman, S.P., L.C. Becker, D.A. Kass, et al. "L-Arginine Therapy in Acute Myocardial Infarction, The Vascular Interaction with Age in Myocardial Infarction (VINTAGE MI) Randomized Clinical Trial." *JAMA* 295 (2006): 58–64.

58. Boger, R.H. "Letter to the Editor re: JAMA Article on L-arginine Therapy in Acute Myocardial Infarction." *Altern Med Rev* (June 2006): 91–92.

59. Bednarz, B., T. Jaxa-Chamiec, P. Maciejewski, et al. "Efficacy and Safety of Oral L-arginine in Acute Myocardial Infarction. Results of the Multicenter, Randomized, Double-blind, Placebo-controlled ARAMI Pilot Trial." *Kardiol Pol* 62:5 (2005): 421–427.

60. Sun, T., W.B. Zhou, X.P. Luo, et al. "Oral L-arginine Supplementation in Acute Myocardial Infarction Therapy: A Meta-analysis of Randomized Controlled Trials." *Clin Cardiol* 32:11 (2009): 649–652.

61. Appleton, J. "Arginine: Clinical Potential of a Semi-Essential Amino Acid." *Altern Med Rev* 7:6 (2002): 512–522.

62. Castillo, L., T.E. Chapman, M. Sanchez, et al. "Plasma Arginine and Citrulline Kinetics in Adults Given Adequate and Arginine-free Diets." *Proc Natl Acad Sci U S A* 90 (1993): 7749–7753. Castillo, L., A. Ajami, S. Branch, et al. "Plasma Arginine Kinetics in Adult Man: Response to an Arginine-free Diet." *Metabolism* 43 (1994): 114–122.

63. Wu, G., and C.J. Meininger. "Arginine Nutrition and Cardiovascular Function." *J Nutr* 130 (2000): 2626–2629.

64. Rakoff, J.S., T.M. Siler, Y.N. Sinha, S.S. Yen. "Prolactin and Growth Hormone Release in Response to Sequential Stimulation by Arginine and Synthetic TRF." *J Clin Endocrinol Metab* 37 (1973): 641–644. Palmer, J.P., R.M. Walter, J.W. Ensinck. "Arginine Stimulated Acute Phase of Insulin and Glucagons Secretion. I. In Normal Man." *Diabetes* 24 (1975): 735–740. Imms, F.J., D.R. London, R.L. Neame. "The Secretion of Catecholamines from the Adrenal Gland Following Arginine Infusion in the Rat." *J Physiol* 200 (1969): 55P–56P. Knopf, R.F., J.W. Conn, S.S. Fajans, et al. "Plasma Growth Hormone Response to Intravenous Administration of Amino Acids." *J Clin Endocrinol Metab* 25 (1965): 1140–1144. Merimee, T.J., D.A. Lillicrap, D. Rabinowitz. "Effect of Arginine on Serum-levels of Human Growth-hormone." *Lancet* 2 (1965): 668–670.

65. Brittenden, J., S.D. Heys, J. Ross, et al. "Natural Cytotoxicity in Breast Cancer Patients Receiving Neoadjuvant Chemotherapy: Effects of L-arginine Supplementation." *Eur J Surg Oncol* 20 (1994): 467–472. Brittenden, J., K.G.M. Park, S.D. Heys, et al. "L-Arginine Stimulates Host Defenses in Patients with Breast Cancer." *Surgery* 115 (1994): 205–212.

66. Cooke, J.P., A.H. Singer, P. Tsao, et al. "Antiatherogenic Effects of L-arginine in the Hypercholesterolemic Rabbit." *J Clin Invest* 90 (1992): 1168–1172. Nakaki, T., and R. Kato. "Beneficial Circulatory Effect of L-arginine." *Jpn J Pharmacol* 66 (1994): 167–171.

67. Boger, R.H. "The Emerging Role of Asymmetric Dimethylarginine as a Novel Cardiovascular Risk Factor." *Cardiovasc Res* 59 (2003): 824–833. Saran, R., J.E. Novak, A. Desai, et al. "Impact of Vitamin E on Plasma Asymmetric Dimethylarginine (ADMA) in Chronic Kidney Disease (CKD): A Pilot Study." *Nephrol Dial Transplant* 18 (2003): 2415–2420.

68. Wolf, A., C. Zalpour, G. Theilmeier, et al. "Dietary L-arginine Supplementation Normalizes Platelet Aggregation in Hypercholesterolemic Humans." *J Am Coll Cardiol* 29 (1997): 479–485. Oomen, C.M., M.J. van Erk, E.J. Feskens, et al. "Arginine Intake and Risk of Coronary Heart Disease Mortality in Elderly Men." *Arterioscler Thromb Vasc Biol* 20 (2000): 2134–2139. Wennmalm, A., A. Edlund, E.F. Granstrom, O. Wiklund. "Acute Supplementation with the Nitric Oxide Precursor L-arginine Does Not Improve Cardiovascular Performance in Patients with Hypercholesterolemia." *Atherosclerosis* 118 (1995): 223–231.

69. Tankersley, R.W. "Amino Acid Requirements of Herpes Simplex Virus in Human Cells." *J Bacteriol* 87 (1964): 609–613.

70. Willis, G.C., and S. Fishman. (1955) "Ascorbic Acid Content of Human Arterial Tissue." *Can Med Assoc J* 72 (April 1955): 500–503.

71. Suarna, C., R.T. Dean, J. May, R. Stocker. "Human Atherosclerotic Plaque Contains Both Oxidized Lipids and Relatively Large Amounts of Alpha-tocopherol and Ascorbate." *Arterioscler Thromb Vasc Biol* 15:10 (1995): 1616–1624.

72. Iuchi, T., M. Akaike, T. Mitsui, et al. "Glucocorticoid Excess Induces Superoxide Production in Vascular Endothelial Cells and Elicits Vascular Endothelial Dysfunction." *Circ Res* 92 (2003): 81–87.

73. Clementi, E., G.C. Brown, M. Feelisch. "Persistent Inhibition of Cell Respiration by Nitric Oxide: Crucial Role of S-nitrosylation of Mitochondrial Complex 1 and Protective Action of Glutathione." *Proc Natl Acad Sci U S A* 95 (1998): 7631–7636. Mogi, M., K. Kinpara, A. Kondo, A. Togari. "Involvement of Nitric Oxide and Biopterin in Proinflammatory Cytokine-induced Apoptotic Cell Death in Mouse Osteoblastic Cell Line MC3T3." *Biochem Pharmacol* 58 (1999): 649–654. Bouton, C. "Nitrosative and Oxidative Modulation of Iron Regulatory Proteins." *Cell Mol Life Sci* 55 (1999): 1043–1053. Donnini, S., and M. Ziche. "Constitutive and Inducible Nitric Oxide Synthase: Role in Angiogenesis." *Antioxid Redox Signal* 4 (2002): 817–823.

74. Kirsch, M., H.G. Korth, R. Sustmann, H. de Groot. "The Pathobiochemistry of Nitrogen Dioxide." *Biol Chem* 383 (2002): 389–399. Chaudiere, J., and R. Ferrari-Iliou. "Intracellular Antioxidants: From Chemical to Biochemical Mechanisms." *Food Chem Toxicol* 37 (1999): 949–962. Regoli, F., and G.W. Winston. "Quantification of Total Oxidant Scavenging Capacity of Antioxidants for Peroxynitrite, Peroxyl Radicals, and Hydroxyl Radicals." *Toxicol Appl Pharmacol* 156 (1999): 96–105.

75. Ceriello, A. "New Insights on Oxidative Stress and Diabetic Complications May Lead to a "Causal" Antioxidant Therapy." *Diabetes Care* 26 (2003): 1589–1596. Trujillo, M., and R. Radi. "Peroxynitrite Reaction with the Reduced and the Oxidized Forms of Lipoic Acid: New Insights into the Reaction of Peroxynitrite with Thiols." *Arch Biochem Biophys* 397 (2002): 91–98. Nakagawa, H., E. Sumiki, M. Takusagawa, et al. "Scavengers for Peroxynitrite: Inhibition of Tyrosine Nitration and Oxidation with Tryptamine Derivatives, Alpha-lipoic Acid and Synthetic Compounds." *Chem Pharm Bull* 48 (2000): 261–265. Whiteman, M., H. Tritschler, B. Halliwell. "Protection Against Peroxynitrite-dependent Tyrosine Nitration and Alpha 1-antiproteinase Inactivation by Oxidized and Reduced Lipoic Acid." *FEBS Lett* 379 (1996): 74–76. Packer, L., K. Kraemer, G. Rimbach. "Molecular Aspects of Lipoic Acid in the Prevention of Diabetes Complications." *Nutrition* 17 (2001): 888–895.

76. Schopfer, F., N. Riobo, M.C. Carreras, et al. "Oxidation of Ubiquinol by Peroxynitrite:

Implications for Protection of Mitochondria Against Nitrosative Damage." *Biochem J* 349 (2003): 35–42.

77. Kjoller-Hansen, L., S. Boesgaard, J.B. Laursen, et al. "Importance of Thiols (SH group) in the Cardiovascular System." *Ugeskr Laeger* 155 (1993): 3642–3645. Ferrari, R., C. Ceconi, S. Curello, et al. "Oxygen Free Radicals and Myocardial Damage: Protective Role of Thiol-containing Agents." *Am J Med* 91 (1991): 95S–105S. Cheung, P.Y., W. Wang, R. Schulz. "Glutathione Protects Against Myocardial Ischemia-reperfusion Injury by Detoxifying Peroxynitrite." *J Mol Cell Cardiol* 32 (2000): 1669–1678. Deneke, S.M. "Thiol-based Antioxidants." *Curr Top Cell Regul* 36 (2000): 151–180. Del Corso, A., P.G. Vilardo, M. Cappiello, et al. "Physiological Thiols as Promoters of Glutathione Oxidation and Modifying Agents in Protein S Thiolation." *Arch Biochem Biophys* 397 (2002): 392–398. Ramires, P.R., and L.L. Ji. "Glutathione Supplementation and Training Increases Myocardial Resistance to Ischemia-reperfusion in Vivo." *Am J Physiol Heart Circ Physiol* 281 (2001): H679–H688.

78. Chaudiere, J., and R. Ferrari-Iliou. "Intracellular Antioxidants: From Chemical to Biochemical Mechanisms." *Food Chem Toxicol* 37 (1999): 949–962.

79. McCarty, M.F. "Oxidants Downstream from Superoxide Inhibit Nitric Oxide Production by Vascular Endothelium—A Key Role for Selenium-dependent Enzymes in Vascular Health." *Med Hypotheses* 53 (1999): 315–325.

80. Terao, J., S. Yamaguchi, M. Shirai, et al. "Protection by Quercetin and Quercetin 3-O-beta-D-glucuronide of Peroxynitrite-induced Antioxidant Consumption in Human Plasma Low-density Lipoprotein." *Free Radical Res* 35 (2001): 925–931. Haenen, G.R., J.B. Paquay, R.E. Korthouwer, et al. "Peroxynitrite Scavenging by Flavonoids." *Biochem Biophys Res Commun* 236 (1997): 591–593.

81. Hickey, S., H. Roberts, R.F. Cathcart. "Dynamic Flow." *J Orthomolecular Med* 20:4 (2005): 237–244.

82. O'Brien, K.D., C.E. Alpers, J.E. Hokanson, et al. "Oxidation-specific Epitopes in Human Coronary Atherosclerosis are Not Limited to Oxidized Low-density Lipoprotein." *Circulation* 94:6 (1996): 1216–1225. Westhuyzen, J. "The Oxidation Hypothesis of Atherosclerosis: An Update." *Ann Clin Lab Sci* 27:1 (1997): 1–10. Reaven, P.D., and J.L. Witztum. "Oxidized Low-density Lipoproteins in Atherogenesis: Role of Dietary Modification." *Annu Rev Nutr* 16 (1996): 51–71. Meagher, E., and D.J. Rader. "Antioxidant Therapy and Atherosclerosis: Animal and Human Studies." *Trends Cardiovasc Med* 11:3–4 (2001): 162–165.

Chapter 8: Quenching the Fire

1. Kolchin, I.N., N.P. Maksiutina, P.P. Balanda, et al. "The Cardioprotective Action of Quercetin in Experimental Occlusion and Reperfusion of the Coronary Artery in Dogs." *Farmakol Toksikol* 54 (1991): 20–23.

2. Simon, E., J. Gariepy, A. Cogny, et al. "Erythrocyte, but Not Plasma, Vitamin E Concentration is Associated with Carotid Intima-media Thickening in Asymptomatic Men at Risk for Cardiovascular Disease." *Atherosclerosis* 159 (2001): 193–200. Andreeva-Gateva, P. "Antioxidant Vitamins—Significance for Preventing Cardiovascular Diseases. Part 1. Oxidized Low-density Lipoproteins and Atherosclerosis; Antioxidant Dietary Supplementation—Vitamin E." *Vutr Boles* 32 (2000): 11–18. Bolton-Smith, C., M. Woodward, H. Tunstall-Pedoe. "The Scottish Heart Health Study. Dietary Intake by Food Frequency Ques-

tionnaire and Odds Ratios for Coronary Heart Disease Risk. II. The Antioxidant Vitamins and Fibre." *Eur J Clin Nutr* 46 (1992): 85–93. Eichholzer, M., H.B. Stahelin, K.F. Gey. "Inverse Correlation Between Essential Antioxidants in Plasma and Subsequent Risk to Develop Cancer, Ischemic Heart Disease and Stroke Respectively: 12-year Follow-up of the Prospective Basel Study." *EXS* 62 (1992): 398–410. O'Byrne, D., S. Grundy, L. Packer, et al. "Studies of LDL Oxidation Following Alpha-, Gamma-, or Delta-tocotrienyl Acetate Supplementation of Hypercholesterolemic Humans." *Free Radical Biol Med* 29 (2000): 834–845.

3. Knekt, P., R. Jarvinen, A. Reunanen, J. Maatela. "Flavonoid Intake and Coronary Mortality in Finland: A Cohort Study." *Br Med J* 312 (1996): 478–481. Formica, J.V., and W. Regelson. "Review of the Biology of Quercetin and Related Bioflavonoids." *Food Chem Toxicol* 33 (1995): 1061–1080.

4. Davis, D.R., M.D. Epp, H.D. Riordan. "Changes in USDA Food Composition Data for 43 Garden Crops, 1950 to 1999." *J Am Coll Nutr* 23:6 (2004): 669–682.

5. Leonard, S.W., Y. Terasawa, R.V. Farese Jr., M.G. Traber. "Incorporation of Deuterated RRR- or All-rac-alpha-tocopherol in Plasma and Tissues of Alpha-tocopherol Transfer Protein-null Mice." *Am J Clin Nutr* 75:3 (2002): 555–560. Traber, M.G. "Utilization of Vitamin E." *Biofactors* 10:2–3 (1999): 115–120. Chopra, R.K., and H.N. Bhagavan. "Relative Bioavailabilities of Natural and Synthetic Vitamin E Formulations Containing Mixed Tocopherols in Human Subjects." *Int J Vitam Nutr Res* 69:2 (1999): 92–95.

6. Heart Protection Study Collaborative Group. "MRC/BHF Heart Protection Study of Cholesterol Lowering with Simvastatin in 20,536 High-risk Individuals: A Randomised Placebo-controlled Trial." *Lancet* 360:9326 (2002): 7–22. Heart Protection Study Collaborative Group. "MRC/BHF Heart Protection Study of antioxidant vitamin supplementation in 20,536 high-risk individuals: a randomised placebo-controlled trial." *Lancet* 360:9326(2002):23-33.

7. Ghirlanda G., A. Oradei, A. Manto, et al. "Evidence of Plasma CoQ$_{10}$-lowering Effect by HMG-CoA Reductase Inhibitors: A Double-blind, Placebo-controlled Study." *J Clin Pharmacol* 33:3 (1993): 226–229. Watts, G.F., C. Castelluccio, C. Rice-Evans, et al. "Plasma Coenzyme Q (Ubiquinone) Concentrations in Patients Treated with Simvastatin." *J Clin Pathol* 46:11 (1993): 1055–1057.

8. Tolbert, J.A. "Coenzyme Q.sub.10 with HMG-CoA Reductase Inhibitors." U.S. Patent 4,929,437, assigned Merck and Co., Rahway, NJ (1990). Brown, M.S. "Coenzyme Q.sub.10 with HMG-CoA Reductase Inhibitors." U.S. Patent 4,933,165, assigned Merck and Co., Rahway, NJ (1990).

9. Arduini, A., A. Peschechera, P. Carminati. "Method of Preventing or Treating Statin-induced Toxic Effects Using L-carnitine or an Alkanoyl L-carnitine." U.S. Patent 6,245,800, assigned Sigma-Tau, Rome, Italy (2001).

10. Whitaker, J.M. "Citizen Petition to Change the Labelling for All Statin Drugs (Mevacor, Lescol, Pravachol, Zocor, Lipitor, and Advicor) Recommending Use of 100–200 mg per Day of Supplemental Coenzyme Q$_{10}$ (Including Cardiomyopathy and Congestive Heart Failure) to Reduce the Risk of Statin-induced Myopathies." U.S Food and Drug Administration petition, May 24, 2002.

11. Lauridsen, C., H. Engel, A.M. Craig, M.G. Traber. "Relative Bioactivity of Dietary RRR- and All-rac-alpha-tocopheryl Acetates in Swine Assessed with Deuterium-labeled Vitamin E." *J Anim Sci* 80:3 (2002): 702–707.

12. Saldeen, T., D. Li, J.L. Mehta. "Differential Effects of Alpha- and Gamma-tocopherol on Low-density Lipoprotein Oxidation, Superoxide Activity, Platelet Aggregation and Arterial Thrombogenesis." *J Am Coll Cardiol* 34:4 (1999): 1208–1215. Kontush, A., T. Spranger, A. Reich, et al. "Lipophilic Antioxidants in Blood Plasma as Markers of Atherosclerosis: The Role of Alpha-carotene and Gamma-tocopherol." *Atherosclerosis* 144:1 (1999): 117–122. Ziouzenkova, O., B.M. Winklhofer-Roob, H. Puhl, et al. "Lack of Correlation Between the Alpha-tocopherol Content of Plasma and LDL, but High Correlations for Gamma-tocopherol and Carotenoids." *J Lipid Res* 37:9 (1996): 1936–1946. Morton, L.W., N.C. Ward, K.D. Croft, I.B. Puddey. "Evidence for the Nitration of Gamma-tocopherol in Vivo: 5-Nitro-gamma-tocopherol is Elevated in the Plasma of Subjects with Coronary Heart Disease." *Biochem J* 364:Part 3 (2002): 625–628.

13. Jiang Q., I. Elson-Schwab, C. Courtemanche, B.N. Ames. "Gamma-tocopherol and Its Major Metabolite, in Contrast to Alpha-tocopherol, Inhibit Cyclooxygenase Activity in Macrophages and Epithelial Cells." *Proc Natl Acad Sci U S A* 97:21 (2000): 11494–11499.

14. Ohrvall, M., G. Sundlof, B.J. Vessby. "Gamma, But Not Alpha, Tocopherol Levels in Serum are Reduced in Coronary Heart Disease Patients." *Intern Med* 239:2 (1996): 111–117.

15. Handelman, G.J., L. Packer, C.E. Cross. "Destruction of Tocopherols, Carotenoids, and Retinol in Human Plasma by Cigarette Smoke." *Am J Clin Nutr* 63:4 (1996): 559–565. Dietrich, M., G. Block, E.P. Norkus, et al. "Smoking and Exposure to Environmental Tobacco Smoke Decrease Some Plasma Antioxidants and Increase Gamma-tocopherol in Vivo After Adjustment for Dietary Antioxidant Intakes." *Am J Clin Nutr* 77:1 (2003): 160–166.

16. Li, D., T. Saldeen, F. Romeo, J.L. Mehta. "Relative Effects of Alpha- and Gamma-Tocopherol on Low-Density Lipoprotein Oxidation and Superoxide Dismutase and Nitric Oxide Synthase Activity and Protein Expression in Rats." *J Cardiovasc Pharmacol Ther* 4:4 (1999): 219–226.

17. Roberts, L.J., J.A. Oates, M.F. Linton, et al. "The Relationship Between Dose of Vitamin E and Suppression of Oxidative Stress in Humans." *Free Radical Biol Med* 43:10 (2007): 1388–1393.

18. Muntwyler, J., C.H. Hennekens, J.E. Manson, et al. "Vitamin Supplement Use in a Low-risk Population of U.S. Male Physicians and Subsequent Cardiovascular Mortality." *Arch Intern Med* 162:13 (2002): 1472–1476.

19. Simon, J.A. "Combined Vitamin E and Vitamin C Supplement Use and Risk of Cardiovascular Disease Mortality." *Arch Intern Med* 162:22 (2002): Editor's Correspondence.

20. Gaziano, M., and J. Muntwyler. "Combined Vitamin E and Vitamin C Supplement Use and Risk of Cardiovascular Disease Mortality." *Arch Intern Med* 162:22 (2002): In reply, Editor's Correspondence.

Chapter 9: An Infectious Disease?

1. Sutter, M.C. "Lessons for Atherosclerosis Research from Tuberculosis and Peptic Ulcer." *Can Med Assoc J* 152:5 (1995): 667–670. Capron, L. "Viruses and Atherosclerosis." Rev Prat 40:24 (1990): 2227–2233. Benitez, R.M. "Atherosclerosis: An Infectious Disease?" *Hosp Pract (Minneap)* 34:9 (1999): 79–82, 85–86, 89–90. Streblow, D.N., S.L. Orloff, J.A. Nelson. "Do Pathogens Accelerate Atherosclerosis?" *J Nutr* 131:10 (2001): 2798S–2804S.

2. Hunter, G.C., A.M. Henderson, A. Westerband, et al. "The Contribution of Inducible

Nitric Oxide and Cytomegalovirus to the Stability of Complex Carotid Plaque." *J Vasc Surg* 30:1 (1999): 36–49. Zhou, Y.F., M. Shou, E. Guetta, et al. "Cytomegalovirus Infection of Rats Increases the Neointimal Response to Vascular Injury Without Consistent Evidence of Direct Infection of the Vascular Wall." *Circulation* 100:14 (1999): 1569–1575.

3. Mehta, J.L., T.G. Saldeen, K. Rand. "Interactive Role of Infection, Inflammation and Traditional Risk Factors in Atherosclerosis and Coronary Artery Disease." *J Am Coll Cardiol* 31:6 (1998): 1217–1225. Broxmeyer, L. "Heart Disease: The Greatest 'Risk' Factor of Them All." *Med Hypotheses* 62:5 (2004): 773–779.

4. Ismail, A., H. Khosravi, H. Olson. "The Role of Infection in Atherosclerosis and Coronary Artery Disease: A New Therapeutic Target." *Heart Dis* 1:4 (1999): 233–240. Kis, Z., K. Burian, D. Virok. et al. "Chronic Infections and Atherosclerosis." *Acta Microbiol Immunol Hung* 48:3–4 (2001): 497–510.

5. Friedman, H.M., E.J. Macarak, R.R. MacGregor, et al. "Virus Infection of Endothelial Cells." *J Infect Dis* 143:2 (1981): 266–273. Tumilowicz, J.J., M.E. Gawlik, B.B. Powell, J.J. Trentin. "Replication of Cytomegalovirus in Human Arterial Smooth Muscle Cells." *J Virol* 56:3 (1985): 839–845. Morre, S.A., W. Stooker, W.K. Lagrand, et al. (2000) "Microorganisms in the Aetiology of Atherosclerosis." *J Clin Pathol* 53:9 (2000): 647–654.

6. Ooboshi , H., C.D. Rios, Y. Chu, et al. "Augmented Adenovirus-mediated Gene Transfer to Atherosclerotic Vessels." *Arterioscler Thromb Vasc Biol* 17:9 (1997): 1786–1792.

7. Ellis, R.W. "Infection and Coronary Heart Disease." *J Med Microbiol* 46:7 (1997): 535–539. Mattila, K.J., V.V. Valtonen, M.S. Nieminen, S. Asikainen. "Role of Infection as a Risk Factor for Atherosclerosis, Myocardial Infarction, and Stroke." *Clin Infect Dis* 26:3 (1998): 719–734.

8. Chiu, B. "Multiple Infections in Carotid Atherosclerotic Plaques." *Am Heart J* 138:5 Part 2 (1999): S534–S536. Vercellotti, G.M. "Overview of Infections and Cardiovascular Diseases." *J Allergy Clin Immunol* 108:4 Suppl (2001): S117–S120.

9. Wanishsawad, C., Y.F. Zhou, S.E. Epstein. "*Chlamydia pneumoniae*–induced Transactivation of the Major Immediate Early Promoter of Cytomegalovirus: Potential Synergy of Infectious Agents in the Pathogenesis of Atherosclerosis." *J Infect Dis* 181:2 (2000): 787–790. Burnett, M.S., C.A. Gaydos, G.E. Madico, et al. "Atherosclerosis in apoE Knockout Mice Infected with Multiple Pathogens." *J Infect Dis* 183:2 (2001): 226–231. Watt, S., B. Aesch, P. Lanotte, et al. "Viral and Bacterial DNA in Carotid Atherosclerotic Lesions." *Eur J Clin Microbiol Infect Dis* 22:2 (2003): 99–105. Virok, D., Z. Kis, L. Kari, et al. "*Chlamydophila pneumoniae* and Human Cytomegalovirus in Atherosclerotic Carotid Plaques—Combined Presence and Possible Interactions." *Acta Microbiol Immunol Hung* 53:1 (2006): 35–50.

10. Armitage, G.C. "Periodontal Infections and Cardiovascular Disease—How Strong is the Association?" *Oral Dis* 6:6 (2000): 335–350.

11. Espinola-Klein, C., H.J. Rupprecht, S. Blankenberg, et al. "Impact of Infectious Burden on Extent and Long-term Prognosis of Atherosclerosis." *Circulation* 105:1 (2002): 15–21. Espinola-Klein, C., H.J. Rupprecht, S. Blankenberg, et al. "Impact of Infectious Burden on Progression of Carotid Atherosclerosis." *Stroke* 33:11 (2002): 2581–2586. Auer, J., M. Leitinger, R. Berent, et al. "Influenza A and B IgG Seroalositivity and Coronary Atherosclerosis Assessed by Angiography." *Heart Dis* 4:6 (2002): 349–354.

12. Speir, E. "Cytomegalovirus Gene Regulation by Reactive Oxygen Species. Agents in Atherosclerosis." *Ann N Y Acad Sci* 899 (2000): 363–374.

13. Daus, H., C. Ozbek, D. Saage, et al. "Lack of Evidence for a Pathogenic Role of *Chlamydia pneumoniae* and Cytomegalovirus Infection in Coronary Atheroma Formation." *Cardiology* 90:2 (1998): 83–88.

14. Epstein, S.E., Y.F. Zhou, J. Zhu. "Infection and Atherosclerosis: Emerging Mechanistic Paradigms." *Circulation* 100:4 (1999): e20–e28.

15. Fabricant, C.G., J. Fabricant, M.M. Litrenta, C.R. Minick. "Virus-induced Atherosclerosis." *J Exp Med* 148:1 (1978): 335–340.

16. Fabricant, C.G., J. Fabricant, M.M. Litrenta, C.R. Minick. "Virus-induced Atherosclerosis." *J Exp Med* 148:1 (1978): 335–340. Minick, C.R., C.G. Fabricant, J. Fabricant. "Atheroarteriosclerosis Induced by Infection with a Herpesvirus." *Am J Pathol* 96:3 (1979): 673–706. Fabricant, C.G., J. Fabricant, C.R. Minick, M.M. Litrenta. "Herpesvirus-induced Atherosclerosis in Chickens." *Fed Proc* 42:8 (1983): 2476–2479. Hajjar, D.P., D.J. Falcone, C.G. Fabricant, J. Fabricant. "Altered Cholesteryl Ester Cycle is Associated with Lipid Accumulation in Herpesvirus-infected Arterial Smooth Muscle Cells." *J Biol Chem* 260:10 (1985): 6124–6128.

17. Kariuki Njenga, M., and C.A. Dangler. "Endothelial MHC Class II Antigen Expression and Endarteritis Associated with Marek's Disease Virus Infection in Chickens." *Vet Pathol* 32:4 (1995): 403–411.

18. Fabricant, C.G., and J. Fabricant. "Atherosclerosis Induced by Infection with Marek's Disease Herpesvirus in Chickens." *Am Heart J* 138:5 Part 2 (1999): S465–S468.

19. Melnick, J.L., E. Adam, M.E. DeBakey. "Cytomegalovirus and Atherosclerosis." *Arch Immunol Ther Exp (Warsz)* 44:5–6 (1996): 297–302.

20. Hajjar, D.P., C.G. Fabricant, C.R. Minick, J. Fabricant. "Virus-induced Atherosclerosis. Herpesvirus Infection Alters Aortic Cholesterol Metabolism and Accumulation." *Am J Pathol* 122:1 (1986): 62–70. Patrascu, I.V. "Marek's Disease. XVII. Studies on Virus-induced Atherosclerosis." *Virologie* 38:4 (1987): 245–250.

21. Shih, J.C., R. Pyrzak, J.S. Guy. "Discovery of Noninfectious Viral Genes Complementary to Marek's Disease Herpes Virus in Quail Susceptible to Cholesterol-induced Atherosclerosis." *J Nutr* 119:2 (1989): 294–298.

22. Span, A.H., G. Grauls, F. Bosman, et al. "Cytomegalovirus Infection Induces Vascular Injury in the Rat." *Atherosclerosis* 93:1–2 (1992): 41–52. Span, A.H., P.M. Frederik, G. Grauls, et al. "CMV-induced Vascular Injury: An Electron-microscopic Study in the Rat." *In Vivo* 7:6A (1993): 567–573.

23. Berencsi, K., V. Endresz, D. Klurfeld, et al. "Early Atherosclerotic Plaques in the Aorta Following Cytomegalovirus Infection of Mice." *Cell Adhes Commun* 5:1 (1998): 39–47. Hsich, E., Y.F. Zhou, B. Paigen, et al. "Cytomegalovirus Infection Increases Development of Atherosclerosis in Apolipoprotein-E Knockout Mice." *Atherosclerosis* 156:1 (2001): 23–28.

24. Benditt, E.P., T. Barrett, J.K. McDougall. "Viruses in the Etiology of Atherosclerosis." *Proc Natl Acad Sci U S A* 80:20 (1983): 6386–6389.

25. Melnick, J.L., E. Adam, M.E. Debakey. "Cytomegalovirus and Atherosclerosis." *Eur Heart J* 14:Suppl K (1993): 30–38. Hendrix, M.G., M.M. Salimans, C.P. van Boven, C.A. Bruggeman. "High Prevalence of Latently Present Cytomegalovirus in Arterial Walls of Patients Suffering from Grade III Atherosclerosis." *Am J Pathol* 136:1 (1990): 23–28. Hendrix, M.G., M. Daemen, C.A. Bruggeman. "Cytomegalovirus Nucleic Acid Distribution

Within the Human Vascular Tree." *Am J Pathol* 138:3 (1991): 563–567. Vercellotti, G.M. "Effects of Viral Activation of the Vessel Wall on Inflammation and Thrombosis." *Blood Coagul Fibrinolysis* 9:Suppl 2 (1998): S3–S6. Hu, W., J. Liu, S. Niu, et al. "Prevalence of CMV in Arterial Walls and Leukocytes in Patients with Atherosclerosis." *Chin Med J (Engl)* 114:11 (2001): 1208–1210.

26. Tanaka, S., Y. Toh, R. Mori, et al. "Possible Role of Cytomegalovirus in the Pathogenesis of Inflammatory Aortic Diseases: A Preliminary Report." *J Vasc Surg* 16:2 (1992): 274–279. Yonemitsu, Y., K. Komori, K. Sueishi, K. Sugimachi. "Possible Role of Cytomegalovirus Infection in the Pathogenesis of Human Vascular Diseases." *Nippon Rinsho* 56:1 (1998): 102–108.

27. Sorlie, P.D., E. Adam, S.L. Melnick, et al. "Cytomegalovirus/Herpesvirus and Carotid Atherosclerosis: The ARIC Study." *J Med Virol* 42:1 (1994): 33–37.

28. Gabrylewicz, B., U. Mazurek, A. Ochala, et al. "Cytomegalovirus Infection in Acute Myocardial Infarction. Is There a Causative Relationship?" *Kardiol Pol* 59:10 (2003): 283–292.

29. Visseren, F.L., K.P. Bouter, M.J. Pon, et al. "Patients with Diabetes Mellitus and Atherosclerosis: A Role for Cytomegalovirus?" *Diabetes Res Clin Pract* 36:1 (1997): 49–55.

30. Melnick, J.L., B.L. Petrie, G.R. Dreesman, et al. "Cytomegalovirus Antigen Within Human Arterial Smooth Muscle Cells." *Lancet* 2:8351 (1983): 644–647. Shih, J.C., and D.W. Kelemen. "Possible Role of Viruses in Atherosclerosis." *Adv Exp Med Biol* 369 (1995): 89–98.

31. Nerheim, P.L., J.L. Meier, M.A. Vasef, et al. "Enhanced Cytomegalovirus Infection in Atherosclerotic Human Blood Vessels." *Am J Pathol* 164:2 (2004): 589–600.

32. Melnick J.L., C. Hu, J. Burek, et al. "Cytomegalovirus DNA in Arterial Walls of Patients with Atherosclerosis." *J Med Virol* 42:2 (1994): 170–174.

33. Hendrix, M.G., P.H. Dormans, P. Kitslaar, et al. "The Presence of Cytomegalovirus Nucleic Acids in Arterial Walls of Atherosclerotic and Nonatherosclerotic Patients." *Am J Pathol* 134:5 (1989): 1151–1157.

34. Biocina, B., I. Husedzinovic, Z. Sutlic, et al. "Cytomegalovirus Disease as a Possible Etiologic Factor for Early Atherosclerosis." *Coll Antropol* 23:2 (1999): 673–681.

35. Cooper, D.K., D. Novitzky, V. Schlegel, et al. "Successful Management of Symptomatic Cytomegalovirus Disease with Ganciclovir After Heart Transplantation." *J Heart Lung Transplant* 10:5 Part 1 (1991): 656–662. Jakel, K.T., T. Loning, R. Arndt, W. Rodiger. "Rejection, Herpesvirus Infection, and Ki-67 Expression in Endomyocardial Biopsy Specimens from Heart Transplant Recipients." *Pathol Res Pract* 188:1–2 (1992): 27–36.

36. Grattan, M.T., C.E. Moreno-Cabral, V.A. Starnes, et al. "Cytomegalovirus Infection is Associated with Cardiac Allograft Rejection and Atherosclerosis." *JAMA* 261:24 (1989): 3561–3566.

37. Loebe, M., S. Schuler, S. Spiegelsberger, et al. "Cytomegalovirus Infection and Coronary Sclerosis After Heart Transplantation." *Dtsch Med Wochenschr* 115:34 (1990): 1266–1269.

38. Adam, E., J.L. Melnick, M.E. DeBakey. "Cytomegalovirus Infection and Atherosclerosis." *Cent Eur J Public Health* 5:3 (1997): 99–106.

39. Olivari, M.T., S.H. Kubo, E.A. Braunlin, et al. "Five-year Experience with Triple-drug

Immunosuppressive Therapy in Cardiac Transplantation." *Circulation* 82:5 Suppl (1990): IV276–IV280.

40. Ventura, H.O., F.W. Smart, D.D. Stapleton, et al. "Cardiac Allograft Vasculopathy: Current Concepts." *J LA State Med Soc* 145:5 (1993): 195–198, 200–202.

41. Pahl, E., F.J. Fricker, J. Armitage, et al. "Coronary Arteriosclerosis in Pediatric Heart Transplant Survivors: Limitation of Long-term Survival." *J Pediatr* 116:2 (1990): 177–183.

42. Yamashiroya, H.M., L. Ghosh, R. Yang, A.L. Robertson Jr. "Herpesviridae in the Coronary Arteries and Aorta of Young Trauma Victims." *Am J Pathol* 130:1 (1988): 71–79.

43. Bruggeman, C.A. "Does Cytomegalovirus Play a Role in Atherosclerosis?" *Herpes* 7:2 (2000): 51–54.

44. Melnick, J.L., E. Adam, M.E. DeBakey. "Cytomegalovirus and Atherosclerosis." *Bioessays* 17:10 (1995): 899–903.

45. Suzuki, S., T. Kimura, K. Ikuta. "Superoxide Generation and Human Cytomegalovirus Infection." *Nippon Rinsho* 56:1 (1998): 75–78. Speir, E., T. Shibutani, Z.X. Yu, et al. "Role of Reactive Oxygen Intermediates in Cytomegalovirus Gene Expression and in the Response of Human Smooth Muscle Cells to Viral Infection." *Circ Res* 79:6 (1996): 1143–1152.

46. Speir, E., Z.X. Yu, V.J. Ferrans, et al. "Aspirin Attenuates Cytomegalovirus Infectivity and Gene Expression Mediated by Cyclooxygenase-2 in Coronary Artery Smooth Muscle Cells." *Circ Res* 83:2 (1998): 210–216.

47. Dhaunsi, G.S., J. Kaur, R.B. Turner. "Role of NADPH Oxidase in Cytomegalovirus-induced Proliferation of Human Coronary Artery Smooth Muscle Cells." *J Biomed Sci* 10:5 (2003): 505–509.

48. Morris-Stiff, G.J., D. Oleesky, W.A. Jurewicz. "Is Selenium Deficiency an Important Risk Factor for Chronic Graft Nephropathy? A Pilot Study." *Transplantation* 76:7 (2003): 1100–1104.

49. Tabib, A., C. Leroux, J.F. Mornex, R. Loire. "Accelerated Coronary Atherosclerosis and Arteriosclerosis in Young Human-immunodeficiency-virus-positive Patients." *Coron Artery Dis* 11:1 (2000): 41–46.

50. Grayston, J.T. "Background and Current Knowledge of *Chlamydia pneumoniae* and Atherosclerosis." *J Infect Dis* 181 (2000): S402–S410.

51. Famularo, G., V. Trinchieri, G. Santini, C. De Simone. "Infections, Atherosclerosis, and Coronary Heart Disease." *Ann Ital Med Int* 15:2 (2000): 144–155. Fong, I.W. "Emerging Relations Between Infectious Diseases and Coronary Artery Disease and Atherosclerosis." *Can Med Assoc J* 163:1 (2000): 49–56. Mussa, F.F., H. Chai, X. Wang, et al. "*Chlamydia pneumoniae* and Vascular Disease: An Update." *J Vasc Surg* 43:6 (2006): 1301–1307.

52. Shi, Y., and O. Tokunaga. "*Chlamydia pneumoniae* and Multiple Infections in the Aorta Contribute to Atherosclerosis." *Pathol Int* 52:12 (2002): 755–763.

53. Kuo, C.C., A.M. Gown, E.P. Benditt, J.T. Grayston. "Detection of *Chlamydia pneumoniae* in Aortic Lesions of Atherosclerosis by Immunocytochemical Stain." *Arterioscler Thromb* 13:10 (1993): 1501–1504. Kuo, C.C., J.T. Grayston, L.A. Campbell, et al. "*Chlamydia pneumoniae* (TWAR) in Coronary Arteries of Young Adults (15–34 Years Old)." *Proc Natl Acad Sci U S A* 92:15 (1995): 6911–6914.

54. Davidson, M., C.C. Kuo, J.P. Middaugh, et al. "Confirmed Previous Infection with

Chlamydia pneumoniae (TWAR) and Its Presence in Early Coronary Atherosclerosis." *Circulation* 98:7 (1998): 628–633.

55. Leinonen, M., and P. Saikku. "Infections and Atherosclerosis." *Scand Cardiovasc J* 34:1 (2000): 12–20. Mawhorter, S.D., and M.A. Lauer. "Is Atherosclerosis an Infectious Disease?" *Cleve Clin J Med* 68:5 (2001): 449–458. Rassu, M., S. Cazzavillan, M. Scagnelli, et al. "Demonstration of *Chlamydia pneumoniae* in Atherosclerotic Arteries from Various Vascular Regions." *Atherosclerosis* 158:1 (2001): 73–79.

56. Ossewaarde, J.M., E.J. Feskens, A. De Vries, et al. "*Chlamydia pneumoniae* is a Risk Factor for Coronary Heart Disease in Symptom-free Elderly Men, but *Helicobacter pylori* and Cytomegalovirus are Not." *Epidemiol Infect* 120:1 (1998): 93–99. de Boer, O.J., A.C. van der Wal, A.E. Becker. "Atherosclerosis, Inflammation, and Infection." *J Pathol* 190:3 (2000): 237–243.

57. Jahromi, B.S., M.D. Hill, K. Holmes, et al. "*Chlamydia pneumoniae* and Atherosclerosis Following Carotid Endarterectomy." *Can J Neurol* Sci 30:4 (2003): 333–339.

58. Kuo, C.C., J.T. Grayston, L.A. Campbell, et al. "*Chlamydia pneumoniae* (TWAR) in Coronary Arteries of Young Adults (15 to 35 Years Old)." *Proc Natl Acad Sci U S A* 92 (1995): 6911–6914.

59. Ngeh, J., V. Anand, S. Gupta. "*Chlamydia pneumoniae* and Atherosclerosis—What We Know and What We Don't." *Clin Microbiol Infect* 8:1 (2002): 2–13.

60. Gurfinkel, E. "Link Between Intracellular Pathogens and Cardiovascular Diseases." *Clin Microbiol Infect* 4:Suppl 4 (1998): S33–S36.

61. Haraszthy, V.I., J.J. Zambon, M. Trevisan, et al. "Identification of Periodontal Pathogens in Atheromatous Plaques." *J Periodontol* 71:10 (2000): 1554–1560.

62. Fong, I.W. "Infections and Their Role in Atherosclerotic Vascular Disease." *J Am Dent Assoc* 133:Suppl (2002): 7S–13S.

63. Meurman, J.H., M. Sanz, S.J. Janket. "Oral Health, Atherosclerosis, and Cardiovascular Disease." *Crit Rev Oral Biol Med* 15:6 (2004): 403–413.

64. Khairy, P., S. Rinfret, J.C. Tardif, et al. "Absence of Association Between Infectious Agents and Endothelial Function in Healthy Young Men." *Circulation* 107:15 (2003): 1966–1971.

65. Stassen, F.R., X. Vega-Cordova, I. Vliegen, C.A. Bruggeman. "Immune Activation Following Cytomegalovirus Infection: More Important Than Direct Viral Effects in Cardiovascular Disease?" *J Clin Virol* 35:3 (2006): 349–353.

66. Schussheim, A.E., and V. Fuster. "Antibiotics for Myocardial Infarction? A Possible Role of Infection in Atherogenesis and Acute Coronary Syndromes." *Drugs* 57:3 (1999): 283–291. Gurfinkel, E.P., and G. Bozovich. "Emerging Role of Antibiotics in Atherosclerosis." *Am Heart J* 138:5 Part 2 (1999): S537–S538. Anderson, J.L., and J.B. Muhlestein. "Antibiotic Trials for Coronary Heart Disease." *Tex Heart Inst J* 31:1 (2004): 33–38.

67. Capron, L. "How to Design Vaccination Trials to Prevent Atherosclerosis." *Am Heart J* 138:5 Part 2 (1999): S558–S559.

68. Capron, L., and B. Wyplosz. "The Infection Theory in Atherosclerosis." *Arch Mal Coeur Vaiss* 91:Special No. 5 (1998): 21–26. Vercellotti, G. "Infectious Agents That Play a Role in Atherosclerosis and Vasculopathies. What Are They? What Do We Do About Them?" *Can J Cardiol* 15:Suppl B (1999): 13B–15B.

69. Rubin, R.H. "Prevention and Treatment of Cytomegalovirus Disease in Heart Transplant Patients." *J Heart Lung Transplant* 19:8 (2000): 731–735.

70. Field, A.K. "Human Cytomegalovirus: Challenges, Opportunities and New Drug Development." *Antivir Chem Chemother* 10:5 (1999): 219–232.

71. Griffiths, P.D. "Cytomegalovirus Therapy: Current Constraints and Future Opportunities." *Curr Opin Infect Dis* 14:6 (2001): 765–768.

72. Grahame-Clarke, C. "Human Cytomegalovirus, Endothelial Function and Atherosclerosis." *Herpes* 12:2 (2005): 42–45.

73. Adams, J.S. Hewison, M. "Unexpected actions of vitamin D: new perspectives on the regulation of innate and adaptive immunity." *Nat Clin Pract Endocrinol Metab* 4(2) (2008): 80–90.

Chapter 10: Linus Pauling and Vitamin C

1. Price, K.D., C.S. Price, R.D. Reynolds. "Hyperglycemia-induced Latent Scurvy and Atherosclerosis: The Scorbutic-metaplasia Hypothesis." *Med Hypotheses* 46:2 (1996): 119–129. Clemetson, C.A. "The Key Role of Histamine in the Development of Atherosclerosis and Coronary Heart Disease." *Med Hypotheses* 52:1 (1999): 1–8.

2. Turley, S.D., C.E. West, B.J. Horton. "The Role of Ascorbic Acid in the Regulation of Cholesterol Metabolism and in the Pathogenesis of Atherosclerosis." *Atherosclerosis* 24:1–2 (1976): 1–18.

3. Schwarz, T., C.K. Stoerk, M. Renwick, et al. "Mineralisation of the Coronary Arteries in the Dog." Abstract, American College of Veterinary Radiology, Annual Scientific Meeting, Chicago, Illinois, December 1–5, 1999.

4. Belfield, W.O. "Chronic Subclinical Scurvy and Canine Hip Dysplasia." *Vet Med Small Anim Clin* 71:10 (1976): 1399–1403.

5. Sako, T., T. Takahashi, K. Takehana, et al. "Chlamydial Infection in Canine Atherosclerotic Lesions." *Atherosclerosis* 162:2 (2002): 253–259.

6. Ginzinger, D.G., J.E. Wilson, D. Redenbach, et al. "Diet-Induced Atherosclerosis in the Domestic Cat." *Lab Investig* 77:11 (November 1997): 409–419.

7. Natarajan R., R.G. Gerrity, J.L. Gu, et al. "Role of 12-lipoxygenase and Oxidant Stress in Hyperglycaemia-induced Acceleration of Atherosclerosis in a Diabetic Pig Model." *Diabetologia* 45:1 (2002): 125–133.

8. Attie, A.D., and M.F. Prescott. "The Spontaneously Hypercholesterolemic Pig as an Animal Model for Human Atherosclerosis." *State of the Art, ILAR News* 30:4 (1988).

9. Martinez Del Rio C. "Can Passerines Synthesize Vitamin C?" *The Auk* 114:3 (1997): 513–516.

9. Vink-Nooteboom, M., N.J. Schoemaker, M.J. Kik, et al. "Clinical Diagnosis of Aneurysm of the Right Coronary Artery in a White Cockatoo (*Cacatua alba*)." *J Small Anim Pract* 39:11 (1998): 533–537.

10. Howerd, A.N. "The Baboon in Atherosclerosis Research: Comparison with Other Species and Use in Testing Drugs Affecting Lipid Metabolism." *Adv Exp Med Biol* 67 (1976): 77–87.

11. Prathap, K. "Spontaneous Aortic Lesions in Wild Adult Malaysian Long-tailed Monkeys (*Macaca irus*)." *J Pathol* 110:2 (1973): 135–143.

12. Prathap, K. "Diet-induced Aortic Atherosclerosis in Malaysian Long-tailed Monkeys (*Macaca irus*)." *J Pathol* 115:3 (1975): 163–174.

13. Linsay, S., and I.L. Chaikoff. "Naturally Occurring Atherosclerosis in Non-human Primates." *J Atheroscler Res* 61 (1966): 36–61.

14. Chatterjee, I.A., B.N. Majumder, N. Subramanian. "Synthesis and Some Major Functions of Vitamin C in Animals." *Ann N Y Acad Sci* 258 (1975): 24–47.

15. Toien, O., K.L. Drew, M.L. Chao, M.E. Rice. "Ascorbate Dynamics and Oxygen Consumption During Arousal from Hibernation in Arctic Ground Squirrels." *Am J Physiol Regul Integrat Comp Physiol* 281 (2001): 572–583.

16. Godin, D.V., and D.M. Dahlman. "Effects of Hypercholesterolemia on Tissue Antioxidant Status in Two Species Differing in Susceptibility to Atherosclerosis." *Res Commun Chem Pathol Pharmacol* 79:2 (1993): 151–166.

17. Siow, R.C., H. Sato, D.S. Leake, et al. "Induction of Antioxidant Stress Proteins in Vascular Endothelial and Smooth Muscle Cells: Protective Action of Vitamin C Against Atherogenic Lipoproteins." *Free Radical Res* 31:4 (1999): 309–318. Siow, R.C., J.P. Richards, K.C. Pedley, et al. "Vitamin C Protects Human Vascular Smooth Muscle Cells Against Apoptosis Induced by Moderately Oxidized LDL Containing High Levels of Lipid Hydroperoxides." *Arterioscler Thromb Vasc Biol* 19:10 (1999): 2387–2394.

18. Arroyo, L.H., and R.T. Lee. "Mechanisms of Plaque Rupture: Mechanical and Biologic Interactions." *Cardiovasc Res* 41:2 (1999): 369–375.

19. Nakata, Y., and N. Maeda. "Vulnerable Atherosclerotic Plaque Morphology in Apoprotein E–deficient Mice Unable to Make Ascorbic Acid." *Circulation* 105:12 (2002): 1485–1490.

20. Paterson, J.C. "Capillary Rupture with Intimal Haemorrhage in the Causation of Cerebral Vascular Lesions." *Arch Pathol* 29 (1940): 345–354.

21. Paterson, J.C. "Some Factors in the Causation of Intimal Hemorrhages and in the Precipitation of Coronary Thrombi." *Can Med Assoc J* (February 1941): 114–120.

22. Bartley, W., H.A. Krebs, J.R.P. O'Brien. "Vitamin C Requirement of Human Adults: A Report by the Vitamin C Subcommittee of the Accessory Food Factors Committee and Others." London: Medical Research Committee, 1953.

23. Weindling, P. "Human Guinea Pigs and the Ethics of Experimentation: The *BMJ*'s Correspondent at the Nuremberg Medical Trial." *Br Med J* 313 (1996): 1467–1470.

24. Willis, G.C. "An Experimental Study of the Intimal Ground Substance in Atherosclerosis." *Can Med Assoc J* 69 (1953): 17–22.

25. Koch, R. "Die Atiologie der Tuberkulose." *Berliner Klin Wochenschift* 15 (April 1882): 221–230. First presented at a meeting of the Physiological Society of Berlin, March 24, 1882.

26. Zilva, S.S. "Vitamin C Requirements of the Guinea-pig." *Biochem J* 30:8 (1936): 1419–1429.

27. Banks, R. "The Guinea Pig: Biology, Care, Identification, Nomenclature, Breeding and Genetics." USAMRIID Seminar Series, February 17, 1989.

28. Fernandez, M.L. "Guinea Pigs as Models for Cholesterol and Lipoprotein Metabolism." *J Nutr* 131:1 (2001): 10–20.

29. Sulkin, N.M., and D.F. Sulkin. "Tissue Changes Induced by Marginal Vitamin C Deficiency." *Ann N Y Acad Sci* 258 (1975): 317–228.

30. Rath, M., and L. Pauling. "Immunological Evidence for the Accumulation of Lipoprotein(a) in the Atherosclerotic Lesion of the Hypoascorbemic Guinea Pig." *Proc Natl Acad Sci* 87:23 (December 1990): 9388–9390.

31. Montano, C.E., M.L. Fernandez, D.J. McNamara. "Regulation of Apolipoprotein B Containing Lipoproteins by Vitamin C Level and Dietary Fat Saturation in Guinea Pigs." *Metabolism* 47 (1998): 883–891. Satinder, S., A.K. Sarkar, S. Majumdar, R.N. Chakravari. "Effects of Ascorbic Acid on the Development of Experimental Atherosclerosis." *Indian J Med Res* 86 (1987): 351–360.

32. Yokota, F., Y. Igarashi, R. Suzue. "Hyperlipidemia in Guinea Pigs Induced by Ascorbic Acid Deficiency." *Atherosclerosis* 38 (1981): 249–254.

33. Ginter, E. "Marginal Vitamin C Deficiency, Lipid Metabolism and Atherogenesis." *Adv Lipid Res* 16 (1978): 167–215.

34. Liu, J.F., and Y.W. Le. "Vitamin C Supplementation Restores the Impaired Vitamin E Status of Guinea Pigs Fed Oxidized Frying Oil." *J Nutr* 128 (1998): 116–122.

35. Sharma, P., J. Pramod, P.K. Sharma, et al. "Effect of Vitamin C Administration on Serum and Aortic Lipid Profile of Guinea Pigs." *Indian J Med Res* 87 (1988): 283–287.

36. Ravnskov, U. "A Hypothesis Out-of-date. The Diet-Heart Idea." *J Clin Epidemiol* 55:11 (2002): 1057–1063.

37. Findlay, G. "A Note on Experimental Scurvy in the Rabbit and the Effects of Antenatal Nutrition." *J Pathol Bacteriol* 24 (1921): 454–455.

38. Hayashi, E., J. Yamada, M. Kunitomo, et al. "Fundamental Studies on Physiological and Pharmacological Actions of L-ascorbate 2-sulfate, On the Hypolipidemic and Antiatherosclerotic Effects of L-ascorbate 2-sulfate in Rabbits." *Jpn J Pharmacol* 28:1 (1978): 61–72. Mahfouz, M.M., H. Kawano, F.A. Kummerow. "Effect of Cholesterol-rich Diets With and Without Added Vitamins E and C on the Severity of Atherosclerosis in Rabbits." *Am J Clin Nutr* 66:5 (1997): 1240–1249. Beetens, J.R., M.C. Coene, A. Veheyen, et al. "Vitamin C Increases the Prostacyclin Production and Decreases the Vascular Lesions in Experimental Atherosclerosis in Rabbits." *Prostaglandins* 32:3 (1986): 335–352. Verlangieri, A.J., T.M. Hollis, R.O. Mumma. "Effects of Ascorbic Acid and Its 2-sulfate on Rabbit Aortic Intimal Thickening." *Blood Vessels* 14:3 (1977): 157–174. Finamore, F.J., R.P. Feldman, G.E. Cosgrove. "L-Ascorbic Acid, L-ascorbate 2-sulfate, and Atherogenesis." *Int J Vitamin Nutr Res* 46:3 (1976): 275–285. Sun, Y.P., B.Q. Zhu, R.E. Sievers, et al. "Effects of Antioxidant Vitamins C and E on Atherosclerosis in Lipid-fed Rabbits." *Cardiology* 89:3 (1998): 189–194. Morel, D.W., M. de la Llera-Moya, K.E. Friday. "Treatment of Cholesterol-fed Rabbits with Dietary Vitamins E and C Inhibits Lipoprotein Oxidation but Not Development of Atherosclerosis." *J Nutr* 124:11 (1994): 2123–2130.

39. Altman, R.F., G.M. Schaeffer, C.A. Salles, et al. "Phospholipids Associated with Vitamin C in Experimental Atherosclerosis." *Arzneimittelforschung* 30:4 (1980): 627–630. Tsimikas, S., B.P. Shortal, J.L. Witztum, W. Palinski. "In Vivo Uptake of Radiolabeled MDA2, an Oxidation-specific Monoclonal Antibody, Provides an Accurate Measure of Atherosclerotic Lesions Rich in Oxidized LDL and is Highly Sensitive to Their Regression." *Arterioscler Thromb Vasc Biol* 20:3 (2000): 689–697.

40. Finamore, F.J., R.P. Feldman, L.J. Serrano, G.E. Cosgrove. "L-Ascorbate 2-Sulfate and

Mobilization of Cholesterol from Plaque Deposited in Rabbit Aortas." *Int J Vitamin Nutr Res* 47:1 (1977): 62–67.

41. Braesen, J.H., U. Beisiegel, A. Niendorf. "Probucol Inhibits Not Only the Progression of Atherosclerotic Disease, but Causes a Different Composition of Atherosclerotic Lesions in WHHL-rabbits." *Virchows Arch* 426:2 (1995): 179–188. Lee, J.Y., A.N. Hanna, J.A. Lott, H.M. Sharma. "The Antioxidant and Antiatherogenic Effects of MAK-4 in WHHL Rabbits." *J Altern Complement Med* 2:4 (1996): 463–478. Schwenke, D.C., and S.R. Behr. "Vitamin E Combined with Selenium Inhibits Atherosclerosis in Hypercholesterolemic Rabbits Independently of Effects on Plasma Cholesterol Concentrations." *Circ Res* 83:4 (1998): 366–377.

42. Maeda, N., H. Hagihara, Y. Nakata, et al. "Aortic Wall Damage in Mice Unable to Synthesize Ascorbic Acid." *Proc Natl Acad Sci U S A* 97:2 (2000): 841–846.

43. Crawford, R.S., E.A. Kirk, M.E. Rosenfeld, et al. "Dietary Antioxidants Inhibit Development of Fatty Streak Lesions in the LDL Receptor-deficient Mouse." *Arterioscler Thromb Vasc Biol* 18:9 (1998): 1506–1513.

44. Willis, G.C., A.W. Light, W.S. Cow. "Serial Arteriography in Atherosclerosis." *Can Med Assoc J* 71 (1954): 562–568.

45. Rath, M., and A. Niedzwiecki. "Nutritional Supplement Program Halts Progression of Early Coronary Atherosclerosis Documented by Ultrafast Computed Tomography." *J Appl Nutr* 48 (1996): 68–78.

46. Dwyer, J.H., L.M. Nicholson, A. Shirecore, et al. "Vitamin C Supplement Intake and Progression of Carotid Atherosclerosis, The Los Angeles Atherosclerosis Study." American Heart Association 40th Annual Conference on Cardiovascular Disease Epidemiology and Prevention, La Jolla, California, March 2–3, 2000.

47. Kritchevsky, S.B., T. Shimakawa, G.S. Tell, et al. "Dietary Antioxidants and Carotid Artery Wall Thickness. The ARIC Study. Atherosclerosis Risk in Communities Study." *Circulation* 92:8 (1995): 2142–2150.

48. Wand, P. "A Pilot Study to Ascertain Carotid Artery Status in High-potency Vitamin C Supplement Takers." *Life Extension News,* lef.org; accessed August 19, 2010.

49. Dwyer, J. Personal communication (e-mail) to Dr. Steve Hickey (2002, 2004).

50. Dwyer, J.H., M.J. Paul-Labrador, J. Fan, et al. "Progression of Carotid Intima-media Thickness and Plasma Antioxidants: The Los Angeles Atherosclerosis Study." *Arterioscler Thromb Vasc Biol* 24:2 (2004): 313–319.

51. Tomoda, H., M. Yoshitake, K. Morimoto, N. Aoki. "Possible Prevention of Postangioplasty Restenosis by Ascorbic Acid." *Am J Cardiol* 78:11 (December 1996): 1284–1286.

52. Fang, J.C., S. Kinlay, J. Beltrame, et al. "Effect of Vitamins C and E on Progression of Transplant-associated Arteriosclerosis: A Randomised Trial." *Lancet* 359:9312 (2002): 1108–1113.

53. Salonen, J.T., K. Nyyssonen, R. Salonen, et al. "Antioxidant Supplementation in Atherosclerosis Prevention (ASAP) Study: A Randomized Trial of the Effect of Vitamins E and C on 3-year Progression of Carotid Atherosclerosis." *J Intern Med* 248:5 (2000): 377–386.

54. Salonen, R.M., K. Nyyssonen, J. Kaikkonen, et al. "Six-year Effect of Combined Vitamin C and E Supplementation on Atherosclerotic Progression: The Antioxidant Supplementation in Atherosclerosis Prevention (ASAP) Study." *Circulation* 107:7 (2003): 947–953.

55. Gale, C.R., H.E. Ashurst, H.J. Powers, C.N. Martyn. "Antioxidant Vitamin Status and Carotid Atherosclerosis in the Elderly." *Am J Clin Nutr* 74:3 (2001): 402–408.

56. Lynch, S.M., J.M. Gaziano, B. Frei. "Ascorbic Acid and Atherosclerotic Cardiovascular Disease." *Subcell Biochem (England)* 25 (1996): 331–367. Ness, A.R., J.W. Powles, K.T. Khaw. "Vitamin C and Cardiovascular Disease: A Systematic Review." *J Cardiovasc Risk* 3:6 (1996): 513–521.

57. Langlois, M., D. Duprez, J. Delanghe, et al. "Serum Vitamin C Concentration is Low in Peripheral Arterial Disease and is Associated with Inflammation and Severity of Atherosclerosis." *Circulation* 103:14 (2001): 1863–1868. Gackowski, D., M. Kruszewski, A. Jawien, et al. "Further Evidence That Oxidative Stress May Be a Risk Factor Responsible for the Development of Atherosclerosis." *Free Radical Biol Med* 31:4 (2001): 542–547. Valkonen, M.M., and T. Kuusi. "Vitamin C Prevents the Acute Atherogenic Effects of Passive Smoking." *Free Radical Biol Med* 28:3 (2000): 428–436. Frei, B. "On the Role of Vitamin C and Other Antioxidants in Atherogenesis and Vascular Dysfunction." *Proc Soc Exp Biol Med* 222:3 (1999): 196–204. Wilkinson, I.B., I.L. Megson, H. MacCallum, et al. "Oral Vitamin C Reduces Arterial Stiffness and Platelet Aggregation in Humans." *J Cardiovasc Pharmacol* 34:5 (1999): 690–693. Frei, B. "Cardiovascular Disease and Nutrient Antioxidants: Role of Low-density Lipoprotein Oxidation." *Crit Rev Food Sci Nutr* 35:1–2 (1995): 83–98. Eichholzer, M., H.B. Stahelin, K.F. Gey. "Inverse Correlation Between Essential Antioxidants in Plasma and Subsequent Risk to Develop Cancer, Ischemic Heart Disease and Stroke Respectively: 12-Year Follow-up of the Prospective Basel Study." *EXS* 62 (1992): 398–410.

58. Jacob, R.A. "Vitamin C Nutriture and Risk of Atherosclerotic Heart Disease." *Nutr Rev* 56:11 (1998): 334–337. Ascherio, A., E.B. Rimm, M.A. Hernan, et al. "Relation of Consumption of Vitamin E, Vitamin C, and Carotenoids to Risk for Stroke Among Men in the United States." *Ann Intern Med* 130:12 (1999): 963–970. Mayer-Davis, E.J., J.H. Monaco, J.A. Marshall, et al. "Vitamin C Intake and Cardiovascular Disease Risk Factors in Persons with Non-insulin-dependent Diabetes Mellitus. From the Insulin Resistance Atherosclerosis Study and the San Luis Valley Diabetes Study." *Prev Med* 26:3 (1997): 277–283.

59. Rath, M., and L. Pauling. "Solution to the Puzzle of Human Cardiovascular Disease: Its Primary Dause is Ascorbate Deficiency, Leading to the Deposition of Lipoprotein(a) and Fibrinogen/fibrin in the Vascular Wall." *J Orthomolecular Med* 6 (1991): 125–134. Rath, M., and L. Pauling. "Unified Theory of Human Cardiovascular Disease Leading the Way to the Abolition of this Disease as a Cause for Human Mortality." *Arteriosclerosis* 9 (1989): 579–592.

60. Rath, M., and L. Pauling. "Lipoprotein(a) is a Surrogate for Ascorbate." *Proc Natl Acad Sci* 87 (1990): 6204–6207.

61. Rath, M., and L. Pauling. "Apoprotein(a) is an Adhesive Protein." *J Orthomolecular Med* 6 (1991): 139–143.

62. Pauling, L., and M. Rath. "Prevention and Treatment of Occlusive Cardiovascular Disease with Ascorbate and Substances That Inhibit the Binding of Lipoprotein(a)." U.S. Patent 5,278,189 (1994). Pauling, L., and M. Rath. "Use of Ascorbate and Tranexamic Acid Solution for Organ and Blood Vessel Treatment Prior to Transplantation." U.S. Patent 5,230,996 (1993).

63. Niendorf, A., M. Rath, K. Wolf, et al. "Morphological Detection and Quantification

of Lipoprotein(a) Deposition in Atheromatous Lesions of Human Aorta and Coronary Arteries." *Virchows Arch Pathol Anat* 417 (1990): 105–111.

64. Tsuchihashi, K., and O. Minari. "Lysine Residues Located on the Surface of Human Plasma High-density Lipoprotein Particles." *Biochim Biophys Acta* 752:1 (1983): 10–18. Fong, B.S., P.O. Rodrigues, A.J. Angel. "Characterization of Low-density Lipoprotein Binding to Human Adipocytes and Adipocyte Membranes." *J Biol Chem* 259:16 (1984): 10168–10174.

Chapter 11: Vitamin E

1. Food and Nutrition Board. *Institute of Dietary Reference Intakes for Vitamin C, Vitamin E, Selenium, and Carotenoids*. Washington, DC: Institute of Medicine, National Academies Press, 2000.

2. Hickey, S., and H. Roberts. *Ridiculous Dietary Allowance*. Raleigh, NC: Lulu Press, 2005.

3. Packer, L., S.U. Weber, G. Rimbach. "Molecular Aspects of Alpha-tocotrienol Antioxidant Action and Cell Signalling." *J Nutr* 131:2 (2001): 369S–373S.

4. Khanna, S., S. Roy, H. Ryu, et al. "Molecular Basis of Vitamin E Action: Tocotrienol Modulates 12-Lipoxygenase, a Key Mediator of Glutamate-induced Neurodegeneration." *J Biol Chem* 278:44 (2003): 43508–43515.

5. Shute, E. "The Current Status of Alpha Tocopherol in Cardiovascular Disease." In: Bailey, H. *Vitamin E, Your Key to a Healthy Heart*. New York: ARC Books, 1964.

6. Stephens, N.G., A. Parsons, P.M. Schofield, et al. "Randomised Controlled Trial of Vitamin E in Patients with Coronary Disease: Cambridge Heart Antioxidant Study (CHAOS)." *Lancet* 349 (1996): 781–786. Mitchinson, M.J., N.G. Stephens, A. Parsons, et al. "Mortality in the CHAOS Trial." *Lancet* 353 (1999): 381–382.

7. Losonczy, K.G., T.B. Harris, R.J. Havlik. (1996) "Epidemiology, Vitamin E and Vitamin C Supplement Use and Risk of All-cause and Coronary Heart Disease Mortality in Older Persons: The Established Populations for Epidemiologic Studies of the Elderly." *Am J Clin Nutr* 64:2 (August 1996): 190–196.

8. Rimm, E.B., M.J. Stampfer, A. Ascherio, et al. "Vitamin E Consumption and the Risk of Coronary Heart Disease in Men." *N Engl J Med* 328:20 (1993): 1450–1456. Stampfer, M.J., C.H. Hennekens, J.E. Manson, et al. "Vitamin E Consumption and the Risk of Coronary Disease in Women." *N Engl J Med* 328:20 (1993): 1444–1449.

9. Gey, K.F., and P. Puska. "Plasma Vitamin E and A Inversely Correlated to Mortality from Ischemic Heart Disease in Cross-Cultural Epidemiology." *Ann N Y Acad Sci* 570 (1989): 268–282. Gey, K.E., P. Puska, P. Jordan, U.K. Moyer. "Inverse Correlation Between Plasma Vitamin E and Mortality from Ischemic Heart Disease in Cross-Cultural Epidemiology." *Am J Clin Nutr* 53 (1991): 3265–3345.

10. Bjelakovic, G., D. Nikolova, L.L. Gluud, et al. "Antioxidant Supplements for Prevention of Mortality in Healthy Participants and Patients with Various Diseases." *Cochrane Database Syst Rev* 2 (2008): CD007176.

11. Ong, W.T. "Don't Take That Vitamin!" Pinoy.md; accessed August 21, 2010.

12. Hickey, S., C. Hancke, R. Verkerk, et al. "Study Employed Inappropriate Statistical Analysis." (2008.) http://www.cochranefeedback.com/cf/cda/citation.do?id=9836#9836. In Feedback to: Bjelakovic, G., D. Nikolova, L.L. Gluud, et al. "Antioxidant Supplements for

Prevention of Mortality in Healthy Participants and Patients with Various Diseases." *Cochrane Database Syst Rev* 2 (2008): CD007176.

13. Schuitemaker, G., B. Jonsson, S. Lawson, et al. "Subjective, Selective, and Biased." (2008.) http://www.cochranefeedback.com/cf/cda/citation.do?id=9837#9837. In Feedback to: Bjelakovic, G., D. Nikolova, L.L. Gluud, et al. "Antioxidant Supplements for Prevention of Mortality in Healthy Participants and Patients with Various Diseases." *Cochrane Database Syst Rev* 2 (2008): CD007176.

14. Gerss, J., and W. Köpcke. "The Questionable Association of Vitamin E Supplementation and Mortality—Inconsistent Results of Different Meta-analytic Approaches." *Cell Mol Biol (Noisy-le-grand)* 55:Suppl (2009): OL1111–OL1120.

15. Azzi, A., I. Breyer, M. Feher, et al. "Specific Cellular Responses to Alpha-tocopherol." *J Nutr* 130:7 (2000): 1649–1652. Azzi, A., and A. Stocker. "Vitamin E: Non-antioxidant Roles." *Prog Lipid Res* 39:3 (2000): 231–255.

16. Liu, M., R. Wallin, A. Wallmon, T. Saldeen. "Mixed Tocopherols Have a Stronger Inhibitory Effect on Lipid Peroxidation Than [Alpha]-Tocopherol Alone." *J Cardiovasc Pharmacol* 39:5 (2002): 714–721.

17. Brigelius-Flohe, R., and M.G. Traber. "Vitamin E: Function and Metabolism." *FASEB J* 13:10 (1999): 1145–1155.

18. Handelman, G.J., L.J. Machlin, K. Fitch, et al. "Oral Alpha-tocopherol Supplements Decrease Plasma Gamma-tocopherol Levels in Humans." *J Nutr* 115:6 (1985): 807–813.

19. Ohrvall, M., G. Sundlof, B. Vessby. "Gamma, but Not Alpha, Tocopherol Levels in Serum are Reduced in Coronary Heart Disease Patients." *J Intern Med* 239:2 (1996): 111–117. Saldeen, T., D. Li, J.L. Mehta. "Differential Effects of Alpha- and Gamma-tocopherol on Low-density Lipoprotein Oxidation, Superoxide Activity, Platelet Aggregation and Arterial Thrombogenesis." *J Am Coll Cardiol* 34:4 (1999): 1208–1215.

20. Jiang, Q., S. Christen, M.K. Shigenaga, B.N. Ames. "Gamma-tocopherol, the Major Form of Vitamin E in the U.S. Diet, Deserves More Attention." *Am J Clin Nutr* 74:6 (2001): 714–722. Gysin, R., A. Azzi, T. Visarius. "Gamma-tocopherol Inhibits Human Cancer Cell Cycle Progression and Cell Proliferation by Down-regulation of Cyclins." *FASEB J* 16:14 (2002): 1952–1954.

21. Horwitt, M.K. "The Promotion of Vitamin E." *J Nutr* 116:7 (1986): 1371–1377. Weiser, H., and M. Vecchi. "Stereoisomers of Alpha-Tocopheryl Acetate. II. Biopotencies of All Eight Stereoisomers, Individually or in Mixtures, as Determined by Rat Resorption-Gestation Tests." *Int J Vitamin Nutr Res* 52 (1982): 351–370. Kaneko, K., C. Kiyose, T. Ueda, et al. "Studies of the Metabolism of Alpha-tocopherol Stereoisomers in Rats Using [5-methyl-(14)C]SRR- and RRR-alpha-tocopherol." *J Lipid Res* 41:3 (2000): 357–367.

22. Stone, W.L., I. LeClair, T. Ponder, et al. "Infants Discriminate Between Natural and Synthetic Vitamin E." *Am J Clin Nutr* 77:4 (2003): 899–906.

23. Lauridsen, C., H. Engel, A.M. Craig, M.G. Traber. "Relative Bioactivity of Dietary RRR- and All-rac-alpha-tocopheryl Acetates in Swine Assessed with Deuterium-labeled Vitamin E." *J Animal Sci* 80:3 (2002): 702–707.

24. Weimann, B.J., and H. Weiser. "Functions of Vitamin E in Reproduction and in Prostacyclin and Immunoglobulin Synthesis in Rats." *Am J Clin Nutr* 53:4 Suppl (1991): 1056S–1060S.

25. Newaz, M.A., and N.N. Nawal. "Effect of Gamma-tocotrienol on Blood Pressure, Lipid

Peroxidation and Total Antioxidant Status in Spontaneously Hypertensive Rats (SHR)." *Clin Exp Hypertens* 21:8 (1999): 1297–1313.

26. Theriault, A., J.T. Chao, Q. Wang, et al. "Tocotrienol: A Review of Its Therapeutic Potential." *Clin Biochem* 32:5 (1999): 309–319.

27. Suzuki, Y.J., M. Tsuchiya, S.R. Wassall, et al. "Structural and Dynamic Membrane Properties of Alpha-tocopherol and Alpha-tocotrienol: Implication to the Molecular Mechanism of Their Antioxidant Potency." *Biochemistry* 32:40 (1993): 10692–10699.

28. Serbinova, E., V. Kagan, L. Han D. Packer. "Free Radical Recycling and Intramembrane Mobility in the Antioxidant Properties of Alpha-tocopherol and Alpha-tocotrienol." *Free Radical Biol Med* 10:5 (1991): 263–275. Serbinova, E.A., and L. Packer. "Antioxidant Properties of Alpha-tocopherol and Alpha-tocotrienol." *Methods Enzymol* 234 (1994): 354–366.

29. Hayes, K.C., A. Pronczuk, J.S. Liang. "Differences in the Plasma Transport and Tissue Concentrations of Tocopherols and Tocotrienols: Observations in Humans and Hamsters." *Proc Soc Exp Biol Med* 202:3 (1993): 353–359.

30. Khanna, S., S. Roy, H. Ryu, et al. "Molecular Basis of Vitamin E Action: Tocotrienol Modulates 12-Lipoxygenase, a Key Mediator of Glutamate-induced Neurodegeneration." *J Biol Chem* 278:44 (2003): 43508–43515.

31. Sen, C.K., S. Khanna, S. Roy, L. Packer. "Molecular Basis of Vitamin E Action. Tocotrienol Potently Inhibits Glutamate-induced pp60(c-Src) Kinase Activation and Death of HT4 Neuronal Cells." *J Biol Chem* 275:17 (2000): 13049–13055.

32. Yusoff, K. "Vitamin E in Cardiovascular Disease: Has the Die Been Cast?" *Asia Pacific J Clin Nutr* 11:Suppl (2002): S443–S447.

33. Theriault, A., J.T. Chao, A. Gapor. "Tocotrienol is the Most Effective Vitamin E for Reducing Endothelial Expression of Adhesion Molecules and Adhesion to Monocytes." *Atherosclerosis* 160:1 (2002): 21–30.

34. Noguchi, N., R. Hanyu, A. Nonaka, et al. "Inhibition of THP-1 Cell Adhesion to Endothelial Cells by Alpha-tocopherol and Alpha-tocotrienol is Dependent on Intracellular Concentration of the Antioxidants." *Free Radical Biol Med* 34:12 (2003): 1614–1620. Naito, Y., M. Shimozawa, M. Kuroda, et al. "Tocotrienols Reduce 25-hydroxycholesterol-induced Monocyte-endothelial Cell Interaction by Inhibiting the Surface Expression of Adhesion Molecules." *Atherosclerosis* 180:1 (2005): 19–25.

35. Inokuchi, H., H. Hirokane, T. Tsuzuki, et al. "Anti-angiogenic Activity of Tocotrienol." *Biosci Biotechnol Biochem* 67:7 (2003): 1623–1627.

36. Qureshi, A.A., S.A. Sami, W.A. Salser, F.A. Khan. "Dose-dependent Suppression of Serum Cholesterol by Tocotrienol-rich Fraction (TRF25) of Rice Bran in Hypercholesterolemic Humans." *Atherosclerosis* 161:1 (2002): 199–207. Theriault, A., Q. Wang, A. Gapor, K. Adeli. "Effects of Gamma-tocotrienol on ApoB Synthesis, Degradation, and Secretion in HepG2 Cells." *Arterioscler Thromb Vasc Biol* 19:3 (1999): 704–712. Mustad, V.A., C.A. Smith, P.P. Ruey, et al. "Supplementation with 3 Compositionally Different Tocotrienol Supplements Does Not Improve Cardiovascular Disease Risk Factors in Men and Women with Hypercholesterolemia." *Am J Clin Nutr* 76:6 (2002): 1237–1243. Pearce, B.C., R.A. Parker, M.E. Deason, et al. "Hypocholesterolemic Activity of Synthetic and Natural Tocotrienols." *J Med Chem* 35:20 (1992): 3595–3606. Qureshi, A.A., N. Qureshi, J.J. Wright, et al. "Lowering of Serum Cholesterol in Hypercholesterolemic Humans by

792

6123

733

8341

45312

Tocotrienols (Palmvitee)." *Am J Clin Nutr* 53:4 Suppl (1991): 1021S–1026S. Raederstorff, D., V. Elste, C. Aebischer, P. Weber. "Effect of Either Gamma-Tocotrienol or a Tocotrienol Mixture on the Plasma Lipid Profile in Hamsters." *Ann Nutr Metab* 46 (2002): 17–23. Pearce, B.C., R.A. Parker, M.E. Deason, et al. "Inhibitors of Cholesterol Biosynthesis. 2. Hypocholesterolemic and Antioxidant Activities of Benzopyran and Tetrahydronaphthalene Analogues of the Tocotrienols." *J Med Chem* 37:4 (1994): 526–541.

37. Suarna, C., R.L. Hood, R.T. Dean, R. Stocker. "Comparative Antioxidant Activity of Tocotrienols and Other Natural Lipid-soluble Antioxidants in a Homogeneous System, and in Rat and Human Lipoproteins." *Biochim Biophys Acta* 1166:2–3 (1993): 163–170.

38. Qureshi, A.A., S.A. Sami, W.A. Salser, F.A. Khan. "Synergistic Effect of Tocotrienol-rich Fraction (TRF(25)) of Rice Bran and Lovastatin on Lipid Parameters in Hypercholesterolemic Humans." *J Nutr Biochem* 12:6 (2001): 318–329.

39. Qureshi, A.A., B.A. Bradlow, L. Brace, et al. "Response of Hypercholesterolemic Subjects to Administration of Tocotrienols." *Lipids* 30:12 (1995): 1171–1177.

40. Verlangieri, A.J., and M.K. Bush. "Effects of d-Alpha-tocopherol Supplementation on Experimentally Induced Primate Atherosclerosis." *J Am Coll Nutr* 11 (1992): 131–138. Passwater, R.A. "Reversing Atherosclerosis: An Interview with Dr. Anthony Verlangieri." *Whole Foods* 15:9 (1992): 27–30.

41. Hodis, H.N., W.J. Mack, L. LaBree, et al. "Serial Coronary Angiographic Evidence That Antioxidant Vitamin Intake Reduces Progression of Coronary Artery Atherosclerosis." *JAMA* 273:23 (1995): 1849–1854.

42. DeMaio, S.J., S.B. King, N.J. Lembo, et al. "Vitamin E Supplementation, Plasma Lipids and Incidence of Restenosis After Percutaneous Transluminal Coronary Angioplasty (PTCA)." *J Am Coll Nutr* 11 (1992): 68–73.

43. Nafeeza, M.I., A.G. Norzana, H.L. Jalaluddin, M.T. Gapor. "The Effects of a Tocotrienol-rich Fraction on Experimentally Induced Atherosclerosis in the Aorta of Rabbits." *Malays J Pathol* 23:1 (2001): 17–25.

44. Hasselwander, O., K. Kramer, P.P. Hoppe, et al. "Effects of Feeding Various Tocotrienol Sources on Plasma Lipids and Aortic Atherosclerotic Lesions in Cholesterol-fed Rabbits." *Food Res Int* 35:2 (2002): 245–251.

45. Kooyenga, D.K., M. Geller, T.R. Watkins, M.L. Bierenbaum. "Antioxidant-induced Regression of Carotid Stenosis Over Three Years." Proceedings of the 16th International Congress of Nutrition. Montreal, Canada, 1997. Tomeo, A.C., M. Geller, T.R. Watkins, et al. "Antioxidant Effects of Tocotrienols in Patients with Hyperlipidemia and Carotid Stenosis." *Lipids* 30:12 (1995): 1179–1183.

46. Black, T.M., P. Wang, N. Maeda, R.A. Coleman. "Palm Tocotrienols Protect ApoE[+/−] Mice from Diet-induced Atheroma Formation." *J Nutr* 130:10 (2000): 2420–2426.

47. Qureshi, A.A., W.A. Salser, R. Parmar, E.E. Emeson. "Novel Tocotrienols of Rice Bran Inhibit Atherosclerotic Lesions in C57BL/6 ApoE-deficient Mice." *J Nutr* 131:10 (2001): 2606–2618.

48. Ismail, N.M., N. Abdul Ghafar, K. Jaarin, et al. "Vitamin E and Factors Affecting Atherosclerosis in Rabbits Fed a Cholesterol-rich Diet." *Int J Food Sci Nutr* 51:Suppl (2000): S79–S94.

49. Teoh, M.K., J.M. Chong, J. Mohamed, K.S. Phang. "Protection by Tocotrienols Against Hypercholesterolaemia and Atheroma." *Med J Malaysia* 49:3 (1994): 255–262.

50. Micheletta, F., S. Natoli, M. Misuraca, et al. "Vitamin E Supplementation in Patients With Carotid Atherosclerosis: Reversal of Altered Oxidative Stress Status in Plasma but Not in Plaque." *Arterioscler Thromb Vasc Biol* 24:1 (2004): 136–140.

Chapter 12: No More Fear

1. Shute, W.E. *Vitamin E for Ailing and Healthy Hearts.* New York: Jove Publications, 1999.

2. Stanger, O., B. Fowler, K. Piertzik, et al. "Homocysteine, Folate and Vitamin B_{12} in Neuropsychiatric Diseases: Review and Treatment Recommendations." *Expert Rev Neurother* 9:9 (2009): 1393–1412.

3. Siri, P.W., P. Verhoef, F.J. Kok. "Vitamins B6, B_{12}, and Folate: Association with Plasma Total Homocysteine and Risk of Coronary Atherosclerosis." *J Am Coll Nutr* 17:5 (1998)" 435–441.

4. Allen, L.H. "Causes of Vitamin B_{12} and Folate Deficiency." *Food Nutr Bull* 29:2 Suppl (2008): S20–S34.

5. Food and Nutrition Board, Institute of Medicine. "Vitamin B_{12}." In: *Dietary Reference Intakes: Thiamin, Riboflavin, Niacin, Vitamin B6, Vitamin B_{12}, Pantothenic Acid, Biotin, and Choline.* Washington DC: National Academy Press, 1998, pp. 306–356.

6. Allen, L.H. "How Common is Vitamin B_{12} Deficiency?" *Am J Clin Nutr* 89:2 (2009): 693S–696S.

7. Waring, R.H. "Report on Absorption of Magnesium Sulfate (Epsom Salts) Across the Skin, for Epson Salt Council." Birmingham, England: School of Biosciences, University of Birmingham, 2005.

8. Hoshino, K., K. Ogawa, T. Hishitani, et al. "Optimal Administration Dosage of Magnesium Sulfate for Torsades de Pointes in Children with Long QT Syndrome." *J Am Coll Nutr* 23:5 (2004): 497S–500S.

9. Duley, L., A.M. Gülmezoglu, D.J. Henderson-Smart. "Magnesium Sulphate and Other Anticonvulsants for Women with Preeclampsia." *Cochrane Database Sys Rev* 2 (2003): CD000025.

10. Maier, J.A.M. "Low Magnesium and Atherosclerosis: An Evidence-based Link." *Mol Aspects Med* 24:1–3 (2003): 137–146.

11. Bolland, M.J., A. Avenell, J.A. Baron, et al. "Effect of Calcium Supplements on Risk of Myocardial Infarction and Cardiovascular Events: Meta-analysis." *Br Med J* 341 (2010): c3691.

12. McCarty, M.F. "An Expanded Concept of 'Insurance' Supplementation—Broad-spectrum Protection from Cardiovascular Disease." *Med Hypotheses* 7:10 (1981): 1287–1302.

13. Chan, A.C., C.K. Chow, D. Chiu. "Interaction of Antioxidants and Their Implication in Genetic Anemia." *Proc Soc Exp Biol Med* 222:3 (1999): 274–282.

14. Shih, J.C. "Atherosclerosis in Japanese Quail and the Effect of Lipoic Acid." *Fed Proc* 15, 42:8 (1983): 2494–2497.

15. Shim, K.F., and P. Vohra. "A Review of the Nutrition of Japanese Quail." *World's Poultry Sci J* 40 (1984): 261–274. Ramachandran, V., and G.H. Arscott. "Minimum Vitamin Requirements and Apparent Vitamin Interrelationships for Growth in Japanese Quail (*Coturnix coturnix japonica*)." *Poultry Sci* 53 (1974): 1969–1970.

16. Zhang, W.J., and B. Frei. "Alpha-lipoic Acid Inhibits TNF-alpha-induced NF-kappaB Activation and Adhesion Molecule Expression in Human Aortic Endothelial Cells." *FASEB J* 15 (2001): 2423–2432. Kunt, T., T. Forst, A. Wilhelm, et al. "Alpha-lipoic Acid Reduces Expression of Vascular Cell Adhesion Molecule-1 and Endothelial Adhesion of Human Monocytes After Stimulation with Advanced Glycation End Products." *Clin Sci (Lond)* 96:1 (1999): 75–82. Bierhaus, A., S. Chevion, M. Chevion, et al. "Advanced Glycation End Product–induced Activation of NF-kappaB is Suppressed by Alpha-lipoic Acid in Cultured Endothelial Cells." *Diabetes* 46 (1997): 1481–1490.

17. Heitzer, T., B. Finckh, S. Albers, et al. "Beneficial Effects of Alpha-lipoic Acid and Ascorbic Acid on Endothelium-dependent, Nitric Oxide–mediated Vasodilation in Diabetic Patients: Relation to Parameters of Oxidative Stress." *Free Radical Biol Med* 31 (2001): 53–61. Morcos, M., V. Borcea, B. Isermann, et al. "Effect of Alpha-lipoic Acid on the Progression of Endothelial Cell Damage and Albuminuria in Patients with Diabetes Mellitus: An Exploratory Study." *Diabetes Res Clin Pract* 52 (2001): 175–183.

18. Ying, Z., N. Kherada, B. Farrar, et al. "Lipoic Acid Effects on Established Atherosclerosis." *Life Sci* 86:3–4 (2010): 95–102.

19. Amom, Z., Z. Zakaria, J. Mohamed, et al. "Lipid-lowering Effect of Antioxidant Alpha-lipoic Acid in Experimental Atherosclerosis." *J Clin Biochem Nutr* 43:2 (2008): 88–94.

20. Zhang, W.J., K.E. Bird, T.S. McMillen, et al. "Dietary Alpha-lipoic Acid Supplementation Inhibits Atherosclerotic Lesion Development in Apolipoprotein E–deficient and Apolipoprotein E/Low-density Lipoprotein Receptor–deficient Mice." *Circulation* 117:3 (2008): 421–428.

21. Vodoevich, V.P. "Effect of Lipoic Acid, Biotin and Pyridoxine on Blood Content of Saturated and Unsaturated Fatty Acids in Ischemic Heart Disease and Hypertension." *Vopr Pitan* 5 (1983): 14–16.

22. Achmad, T.H., and G.S. Rao. "Chemotaxis of Human Blood Monocytes Toward Endothelin-1 and the Influence of Calcium Channel Blockers." *Biochem Biophys Res Comm* 189:2 (1992): 994–1000.

23. Kunt, T., T. Forst, A. Wilhelm, et al. "Alpha-lipoic Acid Reduces Expression of Vascular Cell Adhesion Molecule-1 and Endothelial Adhesion of Human Monocytes After Stimulation with Advanced Glycation End Products." *Clin Sci (Lond)* 96:1 (1999): 75–82.

24. Egan, R.W., P.H. Gale, G.C. Beveridge, et al. "Radical Scavenging as the Mechanism for Stimulation of Prostaglandin Cyclooxygenase and Depression of Inflammation by Lipoic Acid and Sodium Iodide." *Prostaglandins* 16:6 (1978): 861–869.

25. Kohler, H.B., B. Huchzermeyer, M. Martin, et al. "TNF-alpha Dependent NF-kappa B Activation in Cultured Canine Keratinocytes is Partly Mediated by Reactive Oxygen Species." *Vet Dermatol* 12:3 (2001): 129–137.

26. Guilia, M. *French Women Don't Get Fat: The Secret of Eating for Pleasure.* New York: Vintage, 2006.

27. Clowe, W. *The Fat Fallacy: The French Diet Secrets to Permanent Weight Loss.* New York: Three Rivers Press, 2003.

28. Frémon, L. "Biological Effects of Resveratrol." *Life Sci* 66:8 (2000): 663–673.

29. Donnelly, L.E., R. Newton, G.E. Kennedy, et al. "Anti-inflammatory Effects of Resveratrol in Lung Epithelial Cells: Molecular Mechanisms." *Am J Physiol Lung Cell Mol Phys-*

iol 287:4 (2004): L774–L783. Pinto, M.C., J.A. Garcia-Barrado, P. Macias. "Resveratrol is a Potent Inhibitor of the Dioxygenase Activity of Lipoxygenase." *J Agric Food Chem* 47:12 (1999): 4842–4846.

30. Carluccio, M.A., L. Siculella, M.A. Ancora, et al. "Olive Oil and Red Wine Antioxidant Polyphenols Inhibit Endothelial Activation: Antiatherogenic Properties of Mediterranean Diet Phytochemicals." *Arterioscler Thromb Vasc Biol* 23:4 (2003): 622–629.

31. Mnjoyan, Z.H., and K. Fujise. "Profound Negative Regulatory Effects by Resveratrol on Vascular Smooth Muscle Cells: A Role of p53–p21(WAF1/CIP1) Pathway." *Biochem Biophys Res Comm* 311:2 (2003): 546–552.

32. Ibid.

33. Kirk, R.I., J.A. Deitch, J.M. Wu, K.M. Lerea. "Resveratrol Decreases Early Signaling Events in Washed Platelets But Has Little Effect on Platalet in Whole Blood." *Blood Cells Mol Dis* 26:2 (2000): 144–150. Pace-Asciak, C.R., S. Hahn, E.P. Diamandis, et al. "The Red Wine Phenolics Trans-resveratrol and Quercetin Block Human Platelet Aggregation and Eicosanoid Synthesis: Implications for Protection Against Coronary Heart Disease." *Clin Chim Acta* 235:2 (1995): 207–219.

34. Walle, T., F. Hsieh, M.H. Delegge, et al. "High Absorption But Very Low Bioavailability of Oral Resveratrol in Humans." *Drug Metab Dispos* 32:12 (2004): 1377–1382.

35. Wenzel, E., and V. Somoza. "Metabolism and Bioavailability of Trans-resveratrol." *Mol Nutr Food Res* 49:5 (2005): 472–481.

36. Richer, S., W. Stiles, C. Thomas. "Molecular Medicine in Ophthalmic Care." *Optometry* 80:12 (2009): 695–701.

37. Ministry of the Environment, Government of Japan. "Minamata Disease: The History and Measures." Tokyo: Japanese Ministry of the Environment, Government of Japan, 2002. Available online at: http://www.env.go.jp/en/chemi/hs/minamata2002/.

38. Tamashiro, H., M. Arakaki, H. Akagi, et al. "Mortality and Survival for Minamata Disease." *Int J Epidemiol* 14:4 (1985): 582–588.

39. Editors. "Mercury: No Need to Panic." *Life Magazine* (January 29, 1971).

40. Melanson, S.F., E.L. Lewandrowski, J.G. Flood, K.B. Lewandrowski. "Measurement of Organochlorines in Commercial Over-the-counter Fish Oil Preparations: Implications for Dietary and Therapeutic Recommendations for Omega-3 Fatty Acids and a Review of the Literature." *Arch Pathol Lab Med* 129:1 (2005): 74–77.

41. Holick, M.F. "High Prevalence of Vitamin D Inadequacy and Implications for Health." *Mayo Clin Proc* 81:3 (2006): 353–373.

42. Levis, S., A. Gomez, C. Jimenez, et al. "Vitamin D Deficiency and Seasonal Variation in an Adult South Florida Population." *J Clin Endocrinol Metab* 90:3 (2005): 1557–1562.

43. Stretch, E. "Rickets Fear as 40 Fresh Cases Found." *Daily Mirror* (November 13, 2010).

Index

ABOUT THE
AUTHORS

Hilary Roberts' doctoral research on the effects of early-life under-nutrition was carried out in the Department of Child Health at the University of Manchester, England. She is co-author, with Steve Hickey, of *Ascorbate: The Science of Vitamin C, Cancer: Nutrition and Survival, Ridiculous Dietary Allowance,* and *The Cancer Breakthrough.*

Steve Hickey received his doctorate in Medical Biophysics from the University of Manchester, England. He is a member of the Institute of Biology (Pharmacology), a Chartered Biologist, and a former member of the British Computer Society. He has published over 100 scientific papers and is the author of *The Vitamin Cure for Migraines* (Basic Health, 2010) and other books on science and health.